THE
BS
OF MY
MS

Making sense
of a disease
that doesn't
make sense

THE
BS
OF MY
MS

**Making sense
of a disease
that doesn't
make sense**

LAURI L. WOLF

LinkUp
Publishing

THE BS OF MY MS
Making sense of a disease that doesn't make sense

ISBN: 978-0-9885780-0-5
Library of Congress Control Number: 2012954081

Written by Lauri L. Wolf
Book design by Nehmen-Kodner: n-kcreative.com
Published and distributed by LinkUp Publishing, St. Louis, Missouri

www.theBSofmyMS.com
LWolf1@Columbus.RR.com
1985 W. Henderson Rd., #130
Columbus, OH 43220

To my children
Frank, Sophia, and Madison

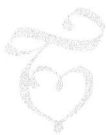

Contents

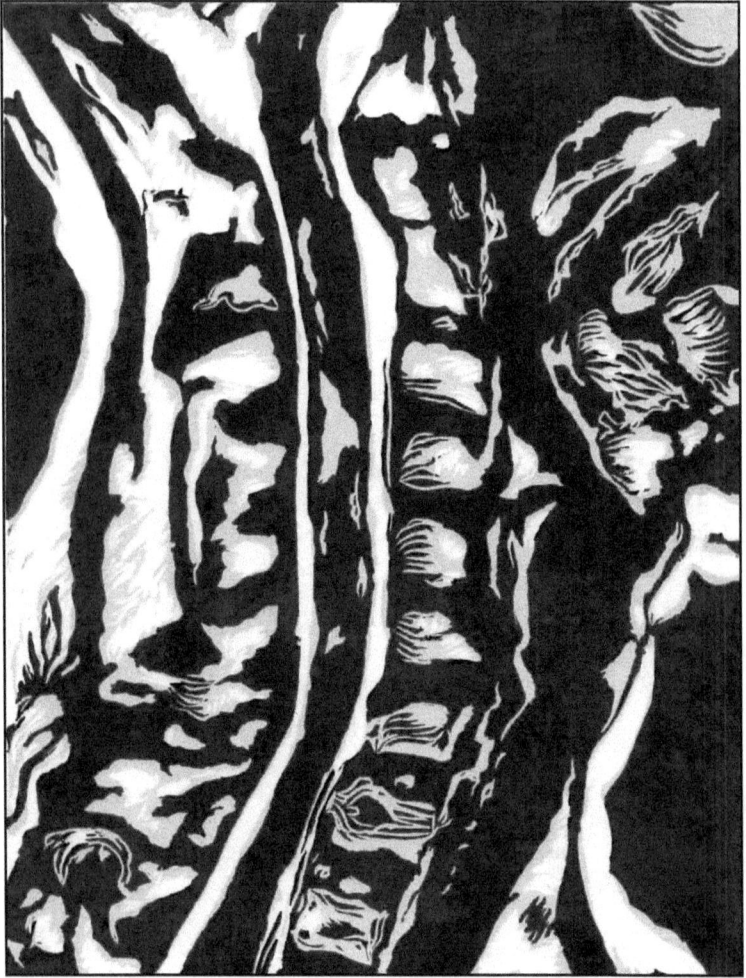

Neurological Ambiguity

Basic relief linoleum print of an MRI image of intricate brain
and spinal cord areas affected by MS

Artwork by Lauri's daughter, Sophia Epitropoulos

Acknowledgments

Thank you to the following who helped make this book a reality: Bobbi Linkemer, my book coach, for her writing finesse and guidance in developing and publishing this book and her astute direction in helping me package my story.

Peggy Nehmen of N-K Creative for her graphic artistry in the design of this book's cover and interior pages.

Sophia Epitropoulos, my oldest daughter, for her creative perspective and artistic contribution at the beginning of this book.

Alice Hohl, president of SiteInsight, and her associates for crafting a functional Web presence and for editing my first, rough draft.

John McCambridge, my physical therapist, for oversight of the written material that pertains to this specialty; more than four years of professional therapy; and a contagious, upbeat spirit he brought to each therapy session.

My personal-care aides for providing their unique styles of physical and emotional caring, compassion, and friendship. Without them, I would not have accomplished nearly as much as I have, both personally and as a parent.

My mother, Dot Gonzalez, for teaching me to cherish the value of each new day and for exemplifying untiring energy.

Carol Wolf, who defies the connotation of the phrase "ex-mother-in-law" and gives it a good name, for giving me the encouragement and confidence to compose my story.

My dear friend, Colette Menhart, for recognizing the intellectual impact of my journey and creating the circumstances necessary to put it on paper.

Posthumous accolades to Jean Dominique Bauby, late author of *The Diving Bell and the Butterfly*, a victim of "locked-in syndrome," who, while only capable of blinking his left eye, poetically and articulately described his conscious world as a prisoner inside a motionless body.

Introduction

MS doesn't define me.
MS is not who I am; it's what I have.

The letters *M* and *S* together represent the acronym for multiple sclerosis. Just this mere abbreviation can evoke apprehension. Because MS is unpredictable and mysterious, it makes people feel uneasy. Most people don't know much about this illness but still shudder and pray it will never strike them. The extent of injury MS causes to the neurological system in one person is unlike what it may do to someone else. Researchers remain baffled, despite six decades of attempting to defeat this assailant and repair its damage.

There is no national registry to accurately identify the affected population, but based on published statistics, the prevalence of MS ranges from 1 in 1,000 to 1 in 1,500 people. Since *everyone* seems to know at least one person with MS, perhaps the incidence is higher than we think. At present, we don't know how MS comes to be, how to prevent it, the number of people who have it, or how to get rid of it. One thing is for certain: People are intrigued by the disease and want to understand it better.

The young woman in the nursing home

My fascination with MS started in 1987 while I was working as a consultant pharmacist for a pharmaceutical-services company in a Springfield, Ohio, nursing home.

I was standing at the nursing station, reviewing resident medical charts, when I caught sight of a young woman who was pushing herself down the hallway in a wheelchair. I stood still and watched her make great effort to hand-power the wheels effectively. She wore a college logo sweatshirt and was obviously younger than the other residents. I wondered why this non-geriatric woman lived in a nursing home.

With each chart I scanned from the rolling chart rack, I examined doctor's orders, lab results, and nursing notes; wrote my own comments; and signed my name in the consultant-pharmacist section. As I focused on the medical cases, my mind kept returning to that young woman and the oddity of a young person living in a nursing home.

Just as I prepared to change nursing stations, this same woman's chart was hand delivered to me by the social services director. The patient was only fifty-three years old and had a diagnosis of MS. I could only remember adrenocorticotropic hormone (ACTH) and high doses of corticosteroids for MS from pharmacy school and previous treatment cases. Her drug orders included only Lioresal (baclofen) to tame muscle spasms and a calcium supplement. Her vitals and blood chemistry were normal. Why wasn't she taking anything to treat her MS?

Unfamiliar with MS at the time, I searched a limited selection of medical reference books in the director of nursing's office (online medical information wasn't the norm circa 1987). Only cortisones were available to treat the symptoms, unlike today when interferons and other drugs are available to suppress the immune system and prevent relapses. Apparently, there was no cure for MS—plain and simple.

This woman's care was puzzling. Why would she live with people thirty-plus years older than she? Why weren't her friends and family helping? Why live in a nursing home where the air was filled with screams of dementia and the odor of urine? I imagined she probably was married to someone who left her because of her illness. Putz.

On the long drive back to Columbus, I couldn't get this young woman off my mind. What would I do if I couldn't take care of myself? I tried not to think about "what if." Then, twelve years later, *I* was diagnosed with MS.

A twist of fate

My lifestyle had been independent and productive before MS toppled it over. "Expect the best but prepare for the worst" became my survival philosophy for coping with shattered dreams and a forced transition into a new reality.

How did this happen? In my mind, I thumbed through a catalog of lifetime activity, wondering what I had done in the past to put myself in position to get MS? Could I have prevented it? Was this a karma thing or punishment from God? Every question was fair game.

Responding to a new diagnosis of MS is no different from responding to any other unexpected, earth-shattering change. "Everyone has her own cross to bear" implies that some sort of suffering plagues each of us. There is no rehearsal opportunity; you can never be "ready" for a disease you will battle for a lifetime. This visitor derailed and overturned my world like an uninvited houseguest who shows up without warning and unpacks a mountain of luggage.

Spending time on anything but figuring out how to deal with my new circumstances was worthless. I looked for material to help me; but while I uncovered plenty of books to explain the science of the disease, I wanted frank, firsthand information from someone who had MS. I had a ton of questions: What could I expect as the disease progressed? What medications worked well? Would I still be a good parent? I could find nothing about how to deal with the physical, psychological, or parenting challenges that come with MS. As the disease morphed, I constantly sought answers to the question, *"Now, what do I do?"*

With so many years of experience with MS, I've realized that explaining what worked or didn't and why might help others manage their MS better. I am also a clinical pharmacist, and though this may sound irrelevant, my knowledge base gives me a unique perspective on managing this disease. I have amassed a great deal of personal experience with medication, and my firsthand knowledge of drug products is valuable.

To give you an understanding of my particular journey, *The BS of my MS: Making sense of a disease that doesn't make sense*, begins by describing an assortment of physical ailments that occurred over the four years prior to my diagnosis but whose source was unclear; the methods specifically used to make a diagnosis of my neurological case; and how the final classification of MS was determined. I then share mischaracterizations of MS, including the observations of others who insisted I looked "too good" to be sick or suggested that I seemed intoxicated because I could not maintain my balance.

I also discuss the following aspects of the disease from the perspective of the patient as well as a professional:

- The importance of examining the validity of alleged MS causes and cures and critically evaluating claims for potential "remedies"
- "Going the distance" to manage bladder, muscle, and a variety of other health problems caused by MS
- Addressing health issues that are not related to MS
- Facing parenting challenges and raising resourceful kids
- Living with the emotional lows
- Prevailing with an optimistic mind-set

My case of MS is uncommon. I have the primary-progressive subtype, which resulted in quadriplegia and a wheelchair. Primary-progressive MS (PPMS) only occurs in about 10 to 15 percent of all MS cases, while the relapsing-remitting subtype (RRMS) occurs in 85 to 90 percent. According to the National MS Society in 2012, approximately 50 percent of all patients with RRMS will evolve into secondary-progressive MS (SPMS) within ten years. I don't talk about managing my disabilities in this book but will cover that topic extensively in my next book, *Moving Right Along*.

MS is a highly misunderstood disease. The front cover of a June 2012 edition of *People* magazine reminded me of that. It featured Sharon Osbourne (wife of heavy metal rock-'n-roll icon Ozzy Osbourne, of Black Sabbath) with their son, Jack, who had just been diagnosed with MS. The headline read, "I Won't Let My Son Die." Sharon has a likable personality on TV shows, and it's easy to empathize with her as a parent who doesn't want to see her child fight an incurable disease. But worrying about death from MS probably should not be a primary concern.

The most common type of MS, relapsing-remitting, can produce spontaneous, surprise interruptions in a person's life for undetermined lengths of time and may later transform into the progressive subtype of the disease. The degree of loss of physical function may require disability assistance, but it rarely results in fatality. A few patients with very severe disability may die prematurely of infectious complications, so that the overall life expectancy is 95 percent of normal.[1]

How can I make a life with MS work for me?

I desperately sought information on how to manage my life with MS; but I couldn't find a single manual written by an individual, rather than an organization, about how to deal with specific physiological, psychological, or parenting challenges for people with this mystifying disease. There simply was no such book; so, I decided to write one.

My story is an account of my personal encounters with the disease. With the exception of the first two chapters, which include my uncertain paths to a diagnosis, the chapters can be read in any order. Here is a synopsis of each chapter to help you find the information you are looking for:

Chapter 1: What Is Wrong with Me?

It took four long years to secure a definitive diagnosis of my slow but steady deterioration. Despite numerous unmistakable signs, ranging from blurry eyesight to weak muscles and early suspicion of MS, an attempt to rule out MS with an MRI was negative for brain lesions. Doctors and friends proposed an amazing array of possible

---

1 National Multiple Sclerosis Society, 2012. (http://www.nationalmssociety.org/
about-multiple-sclerosis/living-with-advanced-ms/prognosis/index.aspx)

causes for my condition, some reasonable, some completely off the mark. I was already losing function in various parts of my body, and I didn't know how fast or how far I would decline.

Chapter 2: My Diagnosis of MS

January 14, 1999, was the great turning point in my life as hallmark signs of MS were identified and confirmed by a neurologist. After countless doctors, MRIs, theories, incorrect diagnoses, tests, and medications, the words were finally uttered aloud: multiple sclerosis. Life as I had known it was over; I was entering an alternate universe, or so it seemed at the time. The physical changes had already begun; it was impossible to predict the emotional fallout that lay ahead.

Chapter 3: MS Causes and Cures: Fact or Fiction?

Despite the fact that little is known about the causes and cures of MS, everyone seems to have an opinion on both. Everything from genetics to Diet Coke has been suggested. What is even more frustrating are the supposed cures, some of which I've actually tried. Frankly, I'm skeptical about any claim for a cure. What it will take is solid scientific research, which is underway but so far has not unraveled this knot.

Chapter 4: MS Misconceptions: Appearances Can Be Deceiving

Considering how difficult it is for doctors to arrive at a definitive diagnosis of MS, it is not so surprising that laymen get it wrong. The symptoms of MS are mysterious, and people can misinterpret what they see. The most common mistake is assuming that I am inebriated because of my unsteady gait or slurred speech, but it doesn't end there. Many disabilities are not obvious; some are completely invisible. The "handicap" placard hanging from our car mirrors is one indication, but few of us pin it to our shirts when we are out and about.

Chapter 5: Juggling Multiple Health Problems with Multiple Sclerosis

Spasticity and bladder problems are common with MS (and are

discussed in detail in separate chapters). Depression, fatigue, and a few other secondary health issues can also be caused by MS. People with MS should realize that they are not immune to other typical adult health problems and should watch for warning signs by checking their blood sugar, blood pressure, cholesterol, immunizations, and a host of markers.

Chapter 6: When the Levee Breaks: Loss of Bladder Control

If we don't know what we have until we lose it, this is certainly true of bladder control. Of all the side effects and symptoms of MS none has been as frustrating and hard to accept as this particular loss. Like other symptoms, it started small; but before long my vocabulary routinely included such terms as *urinary incontinence, self-catheterization,* and *urogynecologist.* I have learned to treat my bladder with the utmost respect.

Chapter 7: Battle Between Brain and Brawn: Spasticity

Spasticity generally refers to stiffness and involuntary muscle spasms and contractions. For those of us with MS, it means much more. Muscle spasticity made all my appendages—legs, arms, hands, and fingers—stiff and noncompliant. My arms and legs often "locked up" and rejected any attempt to straighten or bend them. I tried various therapies and medications over the years until I found one that brought continuous relief from muscle spasms.

Chapter 8: MS Wasn't Enough, Apparently: Trigeminal Neuralgia

Trigeminal neuralgia (TN) is a nerve disorder that causes excruciating, stabbing pain in the face. On a pain measurement scale of one to ten, TN is probably a forty or fifty. Once again, I found myself in the world of medical trial and error. A multitude of procedures were tried, most of which failed, before I was once again a sane, pain-free human being.

Chapter 9: Parenting with MS and Disabilities: Why Not?
There is no law that guarantees parenting rights to a disabled person or assures that he or she will maintain custody of his or her children. In fact, there are many much-publicized cases of mothers who lost custody after bitter court battles. I never wanted to join their ranks. After fourteen years, my kids are doing fine and have learned many important lessons about life.

Chapter 10: Depression, Loneliness, and Fear: Upstream Without a Paddle
We lose many things in life—loved ones, jobs, youth, health—and in each case we grieve. But the loss of *function* is every bit as profound and the grief as painful. With each functional decline, I lost more of the active life I once led, a life that defined my unique persona. One by one, I encountered tasks I had once done with ease that I could no longer do—shop at unique little boutiques, sit at a decent distance from the screen in a movie theater, and even such a small thing as brushing an errant hair off my face.

Chapter 11: Attitude Is Everything: Live, Love, Learn, and Laugh
When I was first diagnosed, I was told that researchers were optimistic about the outlook for MS. That was fourteen years ago. In the meantime, *my* MS continued to progress, unstoppable in its decline. It took a while, but I have developed a tolerant attitude toward my circumstances. An upbeat outlook was essential for my emotional survival. My survival strategy has been to focus on my positive traits, to avert my attention from physical activity I can't do, and to concentrate on things I can, like improving my mental performance.

Feel free to read the chapters in any order you wish. Each one covers a distinct aspect of MS; so, no preceding chapter is necessary to understand any other part of the book. My hope is to reach out to those afflicted with, curious about, or caring for someone with this erratic illness. I want to give a "kindred spirit" the best of what I have learned from the victories, potential potholes, and detours that make up the life of someone with MS.

The way I reacted to having MS is pretty typical, regardless of the specific subtype. Although this book focuses on primary-progressive MS, the information I have shared is meant to inform about all sub-types. My research and personal quest were on finding out how to make my life work. I prayed that my attitude would hold up for the long haul.

Chapter 1
What Is Wrong with Me?

Something was wrong with me, but no one could tell me what it was. It seemed to take forever for doctors to finally confirm that I had MS. Like many other neurological diseases, MS acts in elusive ways; for that reason, it can be difficult to identify. Because the illness plays havoc with the body's electrical system, physiological test results can indicate other problems as well.

Looking back, I had some obvious MS symptoms: I walked with an unsteady gait; my leg and arm muscles were weak; and my speech was randomly slurred. But even after observation and analysis by several doctors, the diagnosis still took years. At the time, no indisputable evidence, such as a blood test or gene marker, existed. Although my current condition would be no different if my MS had been diagnosed years ago, knowing what was happening would have saved me from a ton of frustration and wondering whether my problems were all in my head.

The identification of MS can be tricky, requiring a broad sampling of information and a chronology of somatic events to rule out everything that *isn't* MS; therefore, this is a diagnosis of exclusion. This is particularly true of primary-progressive MS, which might not show the classic lesions found on a brain magnetic resonance imaging (MRI) of patients with relapsing-remitting MS. Lesions from primary-progressive MS are typically found on MRIs of the central nervous system and are located mostly on the spinal cord rather than the brain.

The process of building my clinical diagnosis took a lengthy four years. I had pesky symptoms without any apparent reason. I questioned, wondered, and speculated about what was wrong with me. In my case, MS was eliminated at first as a possible source of my symptoms because the initial MRI of my brain didn't show any lesions. When I continued to demonstrate signs of MS, and the disease could not be ignored as a possible cause, I reluctantly allowed the letters *MS* to be reconsidered as a potential contender.

After I was officially diagnosed with MS, people began to speculate about how I got it and ways I could get rid of it. The ideas were interesting, and some even seemed worth pondering. But with my science background, I realized many hypotheses were illogical and, at times, downright ridiculous. The theories were unsolicited, and it became increasingly difficult to listen politely.

How this whole mess started: tennis lessons and the ophthalmologist

At a family gathering, I casually mentioned to my sister-in-law, Alice, an ophthalmologist, that my vision became blurry in one eye within minutes of any vigorous movement during a tennis lesson. She suggested I make an appointment with her that week.

After the eye assessment in which she couldn't find anything remarkable that might be affecting my eyesight, she handed me the business card of a microphotographer and suggested I contact him for a close-up picture of my eye and retina.

I walked out of her office confident that nothing was wrong because I had passed a comprehensive eye exam, hadn't experienced blurred vision for at least a week, and had a referral if the problems with blurred vision recurred. But that evening, my sister-in-law called to tell me she had made an appointment for me to have an MRI that Friday. I was a little stunned and confused. I paused, struggling to recall her exact words as I left her office. I could have sworn it was, "I want to get a picture of your eye," not "an MRI." An MRI? Wow, this sounds serious, I thought.

"What do you suspect?" I asked. "Well, those *are* signs of MS," she replied with hesitation. "What do you mean by *those*?" I thought I had only complained about blurred vision. "You did say you had tingling in your fingers," she reminded me. I remotely remembered telling her that, but I didn't want to even think she might be right. I *was* experiencing numbness in my fingertips, but it wasn't alarming, just annoying.

"I think you are experiencing Uhthoff's syndrome," she continued. "Your vision becomes blurry when you get overheated, like after exercising. A neuroradiologist colleague suggested you have an MRI."

"Wow. MS? I'm having a hard time putting my arms around this one," I responded.

"Are you kidding? MS? Really?" I did not want an MRI. I could have sworn all I needed was a new pair of contacts. No way, I told myself.

The next afternoon I defiantly called The Ohio State University (OSU) radiology department and canceled the MRI appointment.

Changing my mind about an MRI

Coworkers who were aware of my foggy vision problem were curious to know the results of my eye exam. They were surprised when I mentioned the MS suspicion. As days passed, a few questioned whether my position had changed about doing an MRI. The answer was a definite "No."

A senior executive at the company had a niece who had been recently diagnosed with MS. She and I both had sons about the same age with attention deficit hyperactivity disorder (ADHD). Now, MS had become a topic of conversation. She was obviously disappointed when I told her I had no intention of having an MRI and thoughtfully asked, "What if it's a brain tumor?" I was intrigued. I reconsidered the benefit of an MRI. If it revealed a brain tumor, at least I wouldn't need to deal with MS. I could have the tumor excised, get chemo and maybe some radiation, and be done! I'd also have a justifiable reason for my poor tennis-playing skills. My twisted logic allowed me to view the likelihood of recovering from a brain tumor as better than dealing with a lifetime of MS.

Almost three months had passed since my ophthalmologist had recommended that I have an MRI. I finally rescheduled one at the OSU radiology department.

At the testing site, a radiology technician positioned my body horizontally on a flat surface to roll into an MRI pod. She walked behind a window and activated a switch. As my body was slowly pushed into the tight capsule, I listened to her instructions through the speakers in my headgear.

Claustrophobia and MRIs must be a beastly combination. I can only imagine that those who panic in enclosed spaces would be quick to describe a horrid feeling of asphyxiation inside the machine. Although I did not take anything, I had heard Ativan (lorazepam) and Xanax (alprazolam) have been used to manage severe anxiety attacks for people undergoing an MRI. I found the MRI experience peaceful. I was comfortable in a safe place surrounded by the rumbling sound of jackhammers.

When the test was over, the radiologist and I reviewed dozens of pictures of my brain "slice by slice." The black-and-white films were mounted on a lighted background to illuminate the intricate physiological details of my skull. Thankfully, none displayed any opacity that showed demyelization (damage to the coating of nerve tissue). There was no proof of MS lesions. I exited the radiology building feeling exonerated. Relieved, I convinced myself, "See. I don't have MS."

MS forgotten, reminders ignored

Many warning flags of MS reappeared during the next three years, but I ignored them. I would never voluntarily associate any physical anomaly as a sign of this disease. MS insidiously reveals its presence by short-circuiting muscular coordination. These symptoms made me wonder, was I just plain clumsy, or was it something else? I had a difficult time standing confidently and always felt "off center."

Subconsciously, I must have erased the MS suspicion from my mind. For years, the words never reentered my thoughts. I still had mildly fuzzy vision after hot showers, but because I no longer took tennis lessons, it's hard to say whether playing would have still affected my vision.

Difficulty walking

My sister, Lynette, traveled to the Kentucky Derby every year. In 1996, a year after my eye exam, I joined her and her friends for the RV road trip to Lexington, Kentucky.

We parked on a neighborhood lawn outside the track within reasonable walking distance of the Derby event activities. Since the camper was too cumbersome to drive for local jaunts around town, we walked quite a bit—to the racetrack, to the clubs, and to restaurants. The walking and dancing were affecting me. I was disturbed that I needed to concentrate on keeping my stride and balance with each step, and I couldn't blame it on drinking.

Relationship stress

My first husband was a huge source of stress, which aggravated my MS symptoms, especially in the years before our divorce in 1997. We separated in 1996, and I moved out of the house we shared, hoping that my anxiety would remain behind as well. But like a Pavlovian dog, I became tense, and my heart would palpitate whenever I heard his voice. The cloud of his negativity caused my spasticity to worsen then and for many years to come.

Trouble with balance

One of my best friends, Rosemary, and I organized a champagne tasting with twenty-six female friends. Afterward, we continued the partying at two nightclubs in town. At one of the clubs, a large group of us gathered as girlfriends often do to drink and move to the music. I'm certain I wasn't intoxicated, but standing and dancing were difficult in high-heeled shoes, which hadn't been a problem before. I kicked them off in frustration and rejoined the group in my stocking feet.

Slurred speech

Later that year, during a telephone conversation with a health insurance company executive, I attempted to close our discussion by saying, "Let's talk about this when I'm in Tallahassee." But as I spoke, the words left my mouth at an exaggeratedly slow speed. I sounded drunk. The words seemed to take forever to come out. "Excuse me, one second," I said. Wow, I needed a moment to compose myself. I tried to figure out what the hell had just happened to me. I was shocked and embarrassed, blaming my slurred speech on stress. I took long, deep breaths and returned to the phone to properly finish the conversation.

Sidelined by symptoms

When I began the doctorate program at OSU's College of Pharmacy in the summer of 1997, I parked where most of the students did—in a large parking lot across the street from the college. The walk from my car to the building was about two hundred feet—a long way for someone with difficulty walking. I would silently suffer while staggering from the car to the school. It was now exhausting just to stand erect while walking a straight path. I wondered why it was so difficult to move my body in an upright position.

While I was trying to keep up with classes and homework, I was also managing pharmacy activities full-time for health insurance clients. Normally, my energy level was high and would have allowed me to handle a demanding combination of work and school. But my fatigue was growing, and I needed to withdraw from the academic program.

When visiting Express Scripts' clients in the Southern states, I frequently passed through Atlanta's huge airport, with five large concourses and several smaller ones for regional planes. Flights often land at one concourse, requiring travelers to connect with a plane located at another concourse. Typically, catching a shuttle train and speed walking to the gate for a connecting flight had to be accomplished in less than an hour.

I moved more slowly than normal and constantly turned my head to look back at my wheeled, carry-on luggage to make certain nothing was impeding my speed. I continued to curse the high heels I was wearing. While I waited at the gate of the connecting flight, I would lock my eyes on a Starbucks across a walkway, craving a cappuccino. I grew frustrated knowing that even a seemingly short walk of thirty feet would take everything out of me and probably turn out to be not worth the effort.

Maybe it's depression

My youngest daughter, Madison, was born in January 1998, and during one of her regular newborn checkups, the pediatrician and I chatted as we often did. I asked her what she thought about the problems with my failing muscular strength and walking imbalance. She suggested depression as a possible cause and gave me some Zoloft samples. I thought her idea was plausible and decided an antidepressant was worth a try.

Zoloft therapy turned out to be a huge disappointment. After taking only a couple of doses, I felt like a zombie. I couldn't tolerate the high levels of serotonin the drug caused and decided to continue my search for another therapeutic strategy.

Losing my grip

That summer, my second husband, David, celebrated his thirty-ninth birthday at a popular sports bar. I sat at the bar with him and a friend, drinking a cocktail and smoking a cigarette. Without warning, my extra-thin Capri Ultra Light fell out from between my fingers and rolled onto the floor. The girl sitting next to me appeared startled and gave me one of those "what-the-hell-just-happened" looks. Feeling a little tipsy, I boldly apologized for my inelegance and said, "Tsk. You know, I think I have MS."

Later on at home, David scolded me, "Do *not* tell people you *think* you have MS. You're scaring the hell out of everyone!" Later, recalling this strange incident to others, he snickered, "I told her to stop smoking those skinny little cigarettes and smoke normal-sized ones; then, that wouldn't happen."

That same summer, while standing at the kitchen counter and stirring a pot on the stove, I suddenly dropped to the floor. Why would both of my ankles suddenly give out on me, I wondered.

Can't hold my baby

David's mother flew in from Rhode Island to visit her new granddaughter and our new home. While she stayed at the house with Madison, I decided to visit an internist to discuss the weakness in my legs. I told him how insecure I felt holding my infant baby in one arm while I was moving. He looked at my long, lean body and cocked his head, saying, "You're tall, and your legs are awfully thin. Your body is just now becoming accustomed to the new weight distribution from your pregnancy. You need to increase the strength in your thighs." He demonstrated several squats with his back pressed against a wall. "Stupid me," I thought, "I should have known better. Look at me. I haven't exercised for over a year."

That evening I attempted squats at home and tried to push two four-pound free weights above my head. I wrapped my hands firmly around each and forced them up. As I did, my body listed to one side. No matter how hard I tried, I could not prevent my body from moving off center when I lifted the weights. Ashamed to return to the same internist, I decided to find another physician. I was embarrassed that I couldn't follow through with the simple exercises he had suggested.

Why do I feel unusually helpless carrying my baby?

I continued to struggle with the mundane task of carrying my baby. At less than six months old, Madison weighed no more than my other two children did at the same age, but somehow she seemed heavier. I lacked the confidence to hold her while I was moving around. I clutched her body with one arm and grasped the handrail tightly with the other hand when I walked up and down the stairs. My stride was unsteady. I decided my charade as a sure-footed mother should cease before it put both of us in jeopardy.

Do my shoes fit right?

Why did my shoes not feel right? Forget taking long strides; I only took baby steps from point A to point B. Propelling myself forward on foot moved me only a few inches at a time. Walking and standing straight required total concentration.

Whatever I was wearing—a cocktail dress, wedding dress, formal or casual attire—removing my shoes was becoming my new normal. I had dozens of pairs of shoes, but none of them helped me move any faster or smoother. I gave perfectly good shoes away, yet continued trying on new ones. I was on a quest to find the right fit for me.

Arthritis, perhaps?

While sharing a summer condo that year in New Hampshire, David's father, mentioned that the glucosamine/chondroitin tablets he tried for his arthritis had proved to be disappointingly ineffective. I offered to buy the remainder of his tablets. "Why? Do you have arthritis, too?" he and his wife asked. I briefly explained my physical problems, adding, "No one has been able to put their finger on it yet; but, by the process of elimination, it should be easier to decide what it is." A few months later they traveled to our home in Columbus to visit and asked, "How have the glucosamine tablets been working?"

"You know, I never did end up taking one. I'm thinking my problems might be something unrelated to arthritis," I said.

"Hmm. I bet I know what it is …," my cheeky father-in-law implied that with more lovemaking, I wouldn't have these problems.

This is getting embarrassing

During a trip to visit a client in Baltimore, I walked with a colleague to an open market touted as having the best blue crab cakes in town.

We parked only a short street away and walked on the cobblestone sidewalk. The bumpy, rough surface caused me to take a not-so-elegant fall. The medical director of the health insurance client we had just met with coincidentally was driving on the same street when I took that fateful spill. He yelled out his window and asked whether I needed help. Of all the times! I was embarrassed that he had seen the fall. "Hell yes, I need help!" I thought. But first I needed to find out what was wrong with me so I would know exactly what kind of help I needed. I was a mess and almost ready to give up trying to find out.

Depression again

The second doctor concluded that my physical problems might be related to my emotional ones. "Do you feel depressed?" he asked. I quickly responded, "No, but I'm totally stressed out!"

"Not surprising," he said. "It's so typical of women in your position—taking care of a household and working full-time." This physician's clinical approach caught me off guard. He seemed far more focused on my emotional status than on my physical one. I wasn't expecting it. However, I was willing to consider my emotional state as the root of my physical problems and weighed the antidepressant route once again.

I didn't want a selective serotonin reuptake inhibitor (SSRI) because of my previous experience with Zoloft, so I opted for Wellbutrin SR (bupropion). Wellbutrin has the added benefit of helping with smoking cessation. The drug therapy ran almost nine weeks, adequate time to evaluate its therapeutic effects—for depression at least. I returned to the doctor's office for a follow-up medical visit. He asked me how I was doing with Wellbutrin. With a bit of sarcasm, I answered, "I love Wellbutrin SR and wish to continue its use. But, I still can't walk!" The doctor hesitated for a few moments and said, "I don't think I have any choice but to send you to a neurologist."

Putting two and two together

As I recalled my former sister-in-law's suspicion of MS and thought of my unusual physical symptoms, it jogged my memory of my sister's friend, Rusty. Rusty's father had suffered from relapsing-remitting MS and was in and out of the hospital two to three times each year. Rusty had been riding with her father on his motorcycle when he ran a red light. Rusty asked him whether he could feel his hands on the hand controls, and he said he could not. Recently, I was having difficulty grasping a pair of hair-cutting scissors in my hand. It prompted me to think that her father's symptoms were quite similar to mine. Perhaps I did have MS after all.

When I told Rusty I suspected MS, she gave me a few valuable tips. She strongly suggested I apply for life insurance *before* I got an official diagnosis of MS. Because I had not yet arranged for life insurance with my daughter as beneficiary as I had done for my two older children, I immediately purchased a term life insurance policy before MS could be verified and documented. A diagnosis of MS presented a high risk of financial loss to life insurance companies, and anyone with this condition on his or her health record could typically expect a rejection on a policy application. Rusty's next suggestion was to purchase long-term disability insurance and select the maximum coverage. (It is best to buy disability insurance through an employer because it's less expensive than buying it as an individual.)

Looking back

Since doctors couldn't measure my symptoms the way they could check blood pressure, pulse, or temperature and since extensive reviews by several doctors failed to pinpoint the cause of my illness, in the 1990s, an MS diagnosis seemed to be left to neurologists.

My current condition with MS probably would not be any better had I received an earlier diagnosis, anyway. I have the primary-progressive subtype of MS, which is not responsive to the standard assortment of medications that may have slowed its progression.

After years of failure with immunosuppressive drugs—including Avonex, Copaxone, Novantrone, methylprednisolone, and methotrexate—I was finally diagnosed with primary-progressive MS in

2007, eight years after my initial MS diagnosis in 1999. Knowing that my enigmatic version of MS was a runaway train with no known means of slowing its steady downhill velocity, I finally accepted that I would always need to prepare to be one step ahead of my next physical loss in function.

Chapter 2
My Diagnosis of MS

Years can pass before a multiple sclerosis diagnosis is confirmed. MS symptoms reveal themselves in shadowy ways and vary dramatically from one person to another in terms of physical manifestations, intensity, and rate of progression. Identifying the subtype of MS—relapsing-remitting, secondary-progressive, or primary-progressive can take even longer because observing the symptoms over time is necessary to make a proper determination of how to treat and manage the disease.

The neurologist

It was a long road from my earliest symptoms to a definitive diagnosis of MS. My body experienced an assortment of strange, unexplained physical issues for four years. My ankles unexpectedly caved in while I stood, my right arm felt as if it had "fallen asleep," and my fingers couldn't grasp a pen to write legibly. My brain would send an impulse to an appendage to move, but it either wouldn't or couldn't follow orders. Why? A disconnect between my brain and my body parts was wreaking havoc. I needed to see a neurologist, but my health insurance required an initial work-up by a primary care doctor first.

Between January and October 1998, my balance and strength worsened, but neither of the two internal medicine specialists (primary care doctors) who examined me during that time could figure out what was wrong. The good news was I had finally satisfied the requirement for a referral to a neurological specialist. I had patiently held up my end of the bargain for a year while jumping from one generalist to another seeking an answer. Now, the short six-week wait to see an expert seemed to last forever.

The neurologist to whom I was referred coincidently practiced with the same neurological group I had called on as a pharmaceutical sales representative in the mid-1980s. Twenty years earlier I had promoted an anticonvulsant drug, Mysoline, and a beta-blocker, Inderal, for migraines. The neurologist's familiar face and quiet, gentle demeanor immediately put me at ease. Knowing he was regarded highly by his peers made me feel even more comfortable with my new doctor.

At that first visit the neurologist told me to walk the narrow hallway of his office so he could observe my weak, unsteady gait. He tested my touch sensitivity by lightly poking the skin on the top of my foot and back of my hands. He held my head still and coached my eyes to follow his fingers left to right to test my peripheral visual fields. When he finished, he exited the room.

I sat on his exam table anxiously anticipating his return. To kill time, I scanned the assortment of pamphlets in the wall display and grabbed one titled "Multiple Sclerosis." Minutes later, the doctor reentered the room and fumbled with his papers while preparing to sit on a stool. After a few quiet, awkward moments passed, I snapped the brochure under my chin and announced, "I think it's *this*."

It felt good to blurt out my conclusion because I guess I wanted to hear him say I was right. If I was, maybe I made it easier for him to break the bad news; but, on the other hand, I hoped he would say I was dead wrong. In a casual tone he replied, "Probably is ... but... you'll need to hang in there while we go through what we call 'the million-dollar battery of tests.'"

My second MRI and a VER

The first order of business was an updated MRI and a visual evoked response (VER) test. I needed an MRI for current pictures of my brain; my last one had been four years ago when the ophthalmologist ordered it in 1995. The VER is a test that specifically screens for demyelination diseases, which include MS, Charcot-Marie-Tooth disease, and Devic's disease and are characterized by damaged myelin tissue, which impairs the ability of messages to be transmitted along a nerve.

To conduct the VER test, the technician needed to shave several small areas of hair on my scalp to stick the flat, circular electronic leads to the skin on my head. He instructed me to sit still with my head facing forward, watch a TV monitor, and follow the movement of a spot superimposed over a busy, pulsating geometrical design in the background. The object of the test is to measure the time it takes for the brain to "see" what the eyes are looking at.

The VER evaluates the functioning of the optic nerves and their communication speed to the brain. Although my vision seemed normal, the VER identified problems in the brain that had not been detected by other tests. The test revealed slowed nerve conduction, and although the hesitation was measured by only milliseconds, the findings were consistent with activity in a demyelination disease.

January 14, 1999—diagnosis: MS

There are some days one never forgets. For me, these include the day Kennedy was shot, the explosion of the *Discovery* space shuttle, the collapse of the twin towers at the World Trade Center, and being diagnosed with MS. The moment I heard the words come out of the doctor's mouth, I knew that life as I knew it would never be the same.

The world changed for me after January 14, 1999. My surroundings were the same, but my interpretation of them was different. I viewed some things with hyper vigilance and detail, as if I'd never seen or heard them before. The colors and sounds of other things seemed muted. Although that day continues to fall further away in the chronology of my life, I cling to the era. I talk about events in the 1990s as if they happened yesterday, but my children remind me that those days are now considered "vintage." I apologize to them and others for not honoring the present, but that was the end of one phase of my life and the beginning of another.

I reviewed a letter sent from my ophthalmologist to my neurologist in which she summarized the eye exam she had performed four years earlier. The exam followed my subjective complaints and the subsequent brain MRI, which was negative for lesions. My opthamologist concluded that my diagnosis was Uhthoff's syndrome, or blurred vision with exercise. This was my first clinical symptom of a neurological problem, and it led to my initial MRI, which refuted any suspicion of MS.

Results of my second brain MRI ordered by my neurologist, however, revealed several small opacities on the film that likely indicated demyelination and *probable* MS. My responses to visual stimuli as recorded on the VER test were significantly slower than normal. The poor results of this neurologic exam, in addition to the clinical evaluation conducted by my neurologist, were sufficient for a valid diagnosis of Multiple Sclerosis, ICD-9 (International Classification of Disease, 9th edition) code 340.0—as it is known to the billing departments at doctor's offices and health insurance companies.

David, my second husband, joined me at my neurologist's office for the presentation of his clinical conclusions. The doctor mounted the MRI films on an x-ray projection board and pointed out the tiny lesions on the white tissue of my brain. He continued his talk as if he were sure both David and I were aware of my condition. The doctor was uncomfortable and danced around saying, "You have MS." David's expression showed that he was still unclear about what the doctor was trying to say; so he asked, point blank, "So, is this MS?"

"Yes. It's *probable* MS." The neurologist made a point to include the word *probable* with his diagnosis. For those who can't tolerate vagueness, *probable* is not an acceptable word; but in medical jargon, words such as this were used to indicate the overall uncertainty of a specific disease diagnosis based mostly on clinical rather than hard, measurable data. Words such as *probable* also reduce the physician liability of a wrongful diagnosis. For example, until the 1990s, physicians diagnosed Alzheimer's with the acronym SDAT, or senile dementia of the Alzheimer's type, because it was believed that Alzheimer's could only be diagnosed by an autopsy.

Ironically, part of me was somewhat relieved when I heard the diagnosis. No more suspicions of my creating mysterious muscle complaints and blaming my weak body on simple clumsiness. My physical problems were real and not just in my mind. I was not crazy. I smiled hesitantly when I heard a name assigned to my peculiar condition.

The immediate aftermath of my MS diagnosis

Although David and I left the doctor's office together, as we walked to the car, he stepped up his pace and moved about two or three paces ahead of me. I watched him stride forward and thought, "Oh shit. This is *not* going to be good."

David had already made several challenging transitions out of bachelorhood within a matter of months: He became a husband, a stepfather, and a father. This new development would certainly break him, and I could not bear the guilt and embarrassment of being dependent on him. I feared our relationship would soon and sadly come to an end. I could not imagine having less independence than I already had and relying on him to compensate for what I couldn't do for myself.

While David and I rarely spoke of my MS, he once made the most endearing comment, referring to the future decline we could imagine together—mine from MS and his from too much cigarette smoking. "Don't worry," he said. "When we're both old, we'll live in a house on the Rhode Island shore, and I'll push you around in a wheelchair with my oxygen tank hung on the back." Although David's self-deprecating humor was actually a sad reflection on his cigarette habit, his dry wit came across as funny and quite charming.

We never talked about my MS again.

New neurologist, a twist on my new diagnosis

I wanted to be treated more aggressively and sought a neurologist who specialized in MS at The Ohio State University. My expectations of more refined MS care were unfulfilled. OSU had no "secret cures," and my assigned neurologist surprised me by interpreting my MS subtype differently than I imagined. She defined my history with Uhthoff's syndrome as a relapse event, and any disease progression could be assumed to be secondary (SPMS). I considered my steady deterioration from the start as PPMS.

Cleveland Clinic: "Maybe this is primary progressive"

I visited the Cleveland Clinic Mellen Center for MS for another opinion on my condition. The neurologist there interviewed me for more than an hour. She gathered an impressive, comprehensive history; reviewed the ophthalmologist's report, which had set the diagnostic process into motion; and closely evaluated three MRIs. She thought it was significant that there were no notable changes in my radiological films during the six-year period and boldly stated, "One would never associate your degree of physical disabilities with the results of myelin damage indicated on these MRI films."

The neurologist's insinuation that I had spinal cord lesions not recognized by my brain MRIs could never be verified because having another MRI was contraindicated due to my implanted sacral nerve stimulator for bladder problems (see Chapter 6). Another defining difference of PPMS is that this subtype does not tend to affect cognition the way RRMS and SPMS do. I have an active mind and remain lucid.

Loss of balance and muscle weakness were my initial symptoms and have been referred to as early markers for PPMS. Immunosuppressive medications, the go-to medication for RRMS, failed to control the disease progression throughout my five years of use. Slow physical deterioration developed even years prior to, and a decade after, I received an MS diagnosis.

Nine years after I was first diagnosed with "probable MS," I requested a reevaluation because I wanted my medical record to reflect an accurate MS diagnostic subtype—PPMS.

Why does it take so long to get a diagnosis of MS?

Those experiencing mild MS symptoms may not rush nor describe these events well to a doctor. The physician may need more clinical data because what he or she currently has may be insufficient to make a rightful conclusion. MS is a difficult diagnosis to make. Not long ago, doctors seemed reluctant to label a patient as having MS and seemed to postpone the diagnosis until the patient could barely move a muscle. Then, the announcement, "Gee, I think it's MS" could be assumed to be justified.

Today, the diagnosis of MS has grown to be somewhat more understandable among professionals and laypeople because new medications to slow and control the illness are available. The diagnosis, however, can shake the foundation of one's existence and continues to take a heavy emotional toll on the individual and his or her family.

We now know more about MS

When I phoned my parents to tell them of my diagnosis with MS in 1999, they were mostly silent. Like many others, they had confused MS with the more familiar illness of "Jerry's kids"—muscular dystrophy or MD. They admitted they had no knowledge of this disease. Five or six years later, they announced their surprise at the number of people they subsequently learned had MS.

Now, in the second decade of the 2000s, some believe the number of people with MS is rising. Is this higher number real or perceived? If the number is higher, is it because of people's increased awareness of MS or better diagnostics by physicians? Doctors do seem to be more comfortable with MS as a diagnosis for patients who display quirky neurological symptoms that can't be explained by other diseases. It is also pretty well understood and accepted that people with MS can live long, fruitful lives.

How many people in the United States have MS?

When I was first diagnosed, I scrambled to gather as much information as I could on the subject of MS, including the population affected in the United States. The National Multiple Sclerosis Society claimed about 300,000 to 400,000 people at that time. Fourteen years later, the numbers haven't changed. I contend that the number is actually higher, but there is no accurate registry. The determination of whether someone has MS can be difficult. There are more questions than answers in getting a firm diagnosis. Determining the subtype of MS is even trickier. Typically, it takes years of observation before a patient's subtype can be accurately labeled.

More tests, in addition to the ones I underwent, are becoming available to help confirm the diagnosis of a patient suspected of having the disease. Consequently, patients with MS don't have to live with the uncertainty for as long as I did.

Now that searching for the root of my problems is over, I have mixed feelings about the wait time for my diagnosis. I'm almost glad I didn't know I had MS until four years after I was first suspected of having it. Had I been diagnosed earlier, years of frustration and paranoia that my problems were "mental" would have been eliminated. On the other hand, not knowing what I had turned out to be "ignorant bliss" and gave me a few additional years to enjoy life "as I knew it," rather than focusing on how to prepare for a life controlled by such an ominous, unpredictable disease.

Chapter 3
MS Causes and Cures: Fact or Fiction?

Multiple sclerosis involves deterioration of the myelin sheath that covers the nerve tissue. But despite decades of research, no one has found out what causes MS or how to cure it. The most popular theories are that MS might be caused by the environment, genetics, or a virus.

Is MS genetic?

I'm often asked if MS runs in my family, and my answer is no. Although researchers have not found a genetic link that predisposes a person to MS, it could be that a person's chance of having the disease might be slightly higher than the average person if MS runs in the family.

We all know the huge role genetics plays in the cause of many diseases; so, why not MS?

I wonder whether there is a genetic link to autoimmune diseases in general. For instance, my paternal grandmother had rheumatoid arthritis, and my first cousin has a severe form of psoriasis. These two diseases join MS and others, such as type I diabetes and Crohn's disease, in the autoimmune-disease category. Perhaps the biological influence of two blood relatives with autoimmune diseases put me at a higher risk for having one as well.

Why isn't more research done to find a cure for MS?

MS is the subject of much research, but like the search for answers about many other diseases, sadly, this mystery remains unsolved. Although the physical damage of MS can be tragic, the disease itself is not as common as breast cancer. The average incidence of MS is about one in 1,000,[1] while the chance of a woman having breast cancer in her lifetime, according to the National Cancer Institute, is close to one in eight.[2] I'm inclined to think that a health concern like breast cancer research might deserve priority over MS research[3].

What about environmental toxins and MS?

Environmental toxins are justifiably blamed for provoking an assortment of diseases, but singling out one specific, aggravating agent responsible for MS has never been done.

The community of Wellington, Ohio, has one of the country's highest incidences of MS. It is likely that many of Wellington's residents lived in this industrial part of northern Ohio throughout the 1960s and 1970s. Wellington is also near Lorain, Ohio, which was full of factories at that time and produced untold amounts of polluted air prior to emission-control regulations.

I lived in Lorain from 1962 to 1971 and was exposed to the extremely poor air quality. Before government efforts to rein in pollution, the filthy, sulfur-filled air smelled of rotten eggs and cast a funky yellow-brown haze in the sky. Breathing those gases regularly could not have been healthy for anyone.

The relationship between growing up near this small community with such a high incidence of MS and later developing this disease was hardly surprising. When I recall how rank the environment was at the time, I can't help but wonder whether inhaling those putrid fumes had anything to do with my current condition.

---

1 The epidemiological data for MS is severely out of date. So it is difficult to know the total number of those affected without a permanent, national system. The last national study of incidence and prevalence of MS was conducted in 1975. From the National MS Society to Congress to support the National Neurological Diseases Surveillance System Act on March 22, 2011).

2 National Cancer Institute, National Institutes of Health, http://www.cancer.gov/cancertopics/factsheet/detection/probability-breast-cancerprior.

3 Estimated new cases from breast cancer in the United States in 2012: 226,870 (female); 2,190 (male) and deaths 39,510 (female); 410 (male), National Cancer Institute, http://www.cancer.gov/cancertopics/types/breast

A toxic environment is certainly a suspect for many health problems. But even if there were a master compound that caused MS, is it possible to tease out one element from the composition of pollution as the causative factor?

The challenge of getting reliable information

After my diagnosis of MS was confirmed, it seemed everyone wanted to help fix me. I was inundated with potential healing theories on how to get rid of MS and reasons why I got it in the first place. Those of us who have this disease want solid answers to questions such as, "How do I get rid of it?" Responding with "I don't know," however, is unsettling because no one wants to sound stupid. We all want to say, "I know the answer!" Because of this, people often feel obliged to reply with something plausible. I empathize with people who try to come up with answers or cures for my disease. I know they only want to help, but since my MS is likely to be one of the first topics to come up in conversation with people I meet, it can be frustrating for me. Listening to others try to diagnose or cure my ailments is tiring, especially when I spend much of my time thinking about MS and am probably better informed than the average person.

So, how do we distinguish fact from fiction?

We get our information from newspapers, television, and magazines. We get a lot from casual conversation and idle chitchat. We can find out anything about everything through the Internet, relying heavily on Google or Yahoo! Anything written somehow comes off as truth, and the more desperate we become for answers, the more likely we are to trust unsubstantiated claims.

I'm sure you've heard at least one of these prescriptions for getting rid of hiccups: Put a paper bag over your head and hold your breath; swallow a teaspoon of sugar granules; let someone scare you; have a friend roll up your sleeve to distract you. If a certain method worked to control one person's hiccups, it might be easy to assume that everyone with hiccups would benefit from that method.

Tips for scrutinizing a claim for a cure

I've spent hundreds of hours reading websites, blogs, journals, books, and articles authored by revered researchers and laypeople. So far, I have found no hints of a legitimate cure for MS. I'm skeptical about *any* claim for a cure. Would an announcement as spectacular as a cure for MS be shared with the world through a single person or a chain e-mail? A breakthrough of this magnitude will most likely appear in bold print or be broadcast loudly over the airwaves. Besides the improbable nature of grand scientific news passing through one doubtful source, there are other ways information is packaged that bear scrutiny.

For example, we've all heard the "someone-who-knows-someone" story: "This one guy I know told me about this girl he heard of that did _____ (fill in the blank), and her MS went away." If you have ever participated in a "telephone game" at a party, you know firsthand how the meaning of a simple message can be discombobulated by the time it travels from the first person to the last. Further, the unfettered experience of one person is "anecdotal." Anecdotal information is based on casual observation and cannot be explained systematically. Anecdotal accounts are not necessarily true or false but are unreliable because they are not based on controlled research. The information is cherry-picked and might not be representative of all cases. In other words, it is generalized from an insufficient amount of evidence.

Don't make the mistake of assuming a "recovery" from MS symptoms is a positive response to some external treatment. Recall that the large majority of people with MS (nearly 90 percent) have the relapsing-remitting type, and the unpredictability of the disease can result in someone becoming immobilized from a relapse one day and walking a short time later. In this common type of MS, a natural remission could be interpreted as "healing."

The strength of well-designed scientific studies

A well-informed physician or pharmacist judges a medical treatment not only by the results of studies but also by the overall study design.

For example, the best scientifically sound drug studies are double-blind, randomized, and placebo controlled. *Double-blind* means the patient, as well as the prescriber, is unaware of whether the study drug is being taken. This eliminates the power of suggestion from influencing the study subject as well as the prescriber. *Randomized* refers to an arbitrary selection of individuals, usually picked without the researcher's preference. They are often selected using numbers on a piece of paper with eyes blindfolded or by shaking several dice. *Placebo-controlled* studies include a comparison designed to produce no intentional effect. A placebo could be a sugar pill or no intervention at all for more reliable results.

The power and accuracy of a study are also enhanced when a greater number of research subjects are examined, which are referred to by the letter n. In an anecdotal study the number of study subjects is one, or an n of 1. If MS symptoms disappeared after eating applesauce, but this event occurred in only one person, then (tongue-in-cheek) the results were derived from a very weak study, with an n of 1.

If you want scientific, certifiable proof that "doing something" is better than "not doing something" a proper analysis must be done on the results of the study to determine whether a statistically significant difference exists between the scenarios being compared. Statistical evidence can more accurately determine how typical some things really are. Look for clinical claims where the statistical significance has been tested and evaluated with a resulting p value (which indicates certainty) less than .05. If not, perhaps the claim is making false promises. Remember, *without data it is just an opinion.*

"Scientific" information on the Internet for the cure of MS is as readily available as advertisements for erectile dysfunction treatments. As my father often warned, "You gotta tell shit from Shinola."[4] Be discerning of any advertised claim.

"I-know-how-you-got-and-how-you-can-get-rid-of-MS" stories

The following are well-intended, unproven methods and stories I

---

4 Shinola was a popular brand of men's shoe polish, circa 1930-60

heard that explain how I became afflicted with MS and how I could make it go away. Some people even acted surprised that I hadn't already figured out what they knew and became angry that I had not followed their advice. You may have heard similar stories.

• *The carpenter and Diet Coke*

I commissioned a middle-aged couple who owned a carpentry company to refinish the oak floors of an older home I purchased. After sanding the badly scratched top layer of the wood flooring, the husband turned off his loud floor-refinishing machine, stopped, and wiped his sweaty brow. Just then, he watched me try hard to steady myself as I teetered across the room. From a crouched position, he turned his head to ask me with a Southern drawl, "What's your problem, darlin'?"

"I have MS," I answered candidly with a smile and the same tone I routinely use. I wasn't in the mood to engage in conversation, as I sometimes deliberately tried to avoid patronizing remarks.

He shook his head to stare at me and pursed his lips. I could tell the wheels behind his eyes were turning.

He methodically removed his gloves finger by finger and firmly said with a deadpan tone, "You know what your problem is?" Although it sounded like he had asked me a question, I knew his real intention was to tell me that he knew the answer. I wanted to respond sarcastically, "Gee, I've spent so much time and money on medical professionals, when I only needed to call you!" But, I forced myself to behave and accept his words kindly.

"I seen all them Diet Coke cans you got," he said.

"All them Diet Coke cans" he was referring to was the heap of empty cans loaded in my recycle bins on the driveway waiting for that day's pickup. The large number of empty cans obviously indicated that I routinely consumed aspartame. There was and still is information connecting aspartame with MS, but it is an unproven claim that has been widely broadcast via e-mail and the Internet. Health tragedies from aspartame have become urban legend.

I asked, "Why do all the other Diet Coke drinking people in the world not have MS?" No answer.[5]

• Do bee stings work?

Bee sting therapy has been tried as treatment for some autoimmune diseases but is not supported by any scientific studies that prove it has therapeutic value for MS. Nonetheless, the use of these insects to deliberately pierce the skin and inject their venom as anti-MS therapy has drawn quite a bit of interest.

A member of the church I attend built an apiary in his backyard. He was an intellectual Cornell graduate who took great pride and interest in honeybees and the therapeutic uses of their venom.

I accepted his offer to introduce me to the bee-sting experience. He and his wife and son came to my home with a little mesh cage filled with a half dozen bees, set it on my dining room table, reached inside, and trapped a bee with a small pair of metal tongs.

The three circled around me and closed their eyes in prayer before applying the bee to my flesh. The father then placed the struggling insect on the bare skin of my forearm. The bee quickly stabbed me. Just like a needle and syringe, it injected me with a dose of its toxin. The stinger remained in the skin of my arm for about fifteen minutes before it was removed. According to several websites about bee-sting therapy, patients are advised to repeat this process for approximately three sessions per week, with each session including anywhere from twenty to forty bee stings. My bee venom experience failed to produce any noticeably good result. In fact, the skin on my arm turned red and itchy for several days and caused an overall mild increase in my skin temperature.

The philosophy behind using bee venom is to distract the body's immune system from destroying the myelin tissue and redirect it

---

5 FDA officials describe aspartame as "one of the most thoroughly tested and studied food additives the agency has ever approved" and its safety as "clear cut." John Henkel, "Sugar Substitutes: Americans Opt for Sweetness and Lite," *FDA Consumer Magazine* 33 no. 6 (1999): 12–6. PMID 10628311. Archived from the original on January 2, 2007.

to attack the antigenic activity of the venom responsible for causing irritation and inflammation to the body. Continued Internet searches revealed blogs by plenty of people with MS who wanted to try bee-sting therapy. The bloggers were also looking for others who could share their experiences.

The most detailed information I acquired was from a girl whose urge to urinate was postponed by one to two hours after receiving twenty-nine stings every other day. I could not justify the misery of enduring the pain of more than two dozen bee stings every other day for the insignificant result of *possibly* prolonging the need to use the toilet for only one stinking hour or two.

Using bee venom to ward off the damage caused by MS seemed to have some logic, but I never found it beneficial. I couldn't locate any scientific evidence conducted on bee-sting therapy to back up the hype, nor could I convince myself to continue with bee therapy.

• *Do silver fillings in teeth cause MS?*
Removing the amalgam fillings from your teeth and replacing them with composite fillings was quite the trend for treating and preventing MS. But before going through the discomfort and expense of having every silver filling removed, check the scientific evidence that substantiates whether amalgam fillings are really a legitimate MS issue.

Another frequently repeated rationale for MS is that a trace amount of toxic mercury in amalgam fillings causes the disease. However, there is no substantial proof that mercury toxicity and MS occur with these fillings or that composite fillings protect anyone from getting MS.

A new dentist evaluated my teeth; during the exam, he was surprised that I hadn't been asked by any other dentists to remove my silver fillings and replace them with composite ones. As we spoke further of my MS, he shared news of another patient with MS who underwent this procedure and was quite satisfied. What the dentist failed to realize was that this patient had RRMS, and his condition deteriorated significantly over a three-year period.

During the next ten years, several dental students and two senior dentists also asked whether any other dentist had ever talked with me about amalgam fillings and MS. Although I never made an effort to change the material used as fillings for the cavities in my teeth, I did need to have two old amalgam fillings removed and opted to have them refilled with composite ones for the aesthetic value.

Six years after I replaced them, the new composite fillings contracted and allowed bacteria to creep in through the exposed seams of the tooth. Amalgam fillings normally do not shrink and remain sealed to keep out decay. The two molars with composite fillings developed deep cavities with resulting abscesses. Ultimately, root canals were required on both teeth. It wasn't pleasant.

• *Does stress cause MS?*
A family friend's mother always announces she "knows" my MS was caused by my first ex-husband. However, the stress I experienced during our marriage could never have been tested nor proven to cause my disease.

My gut belief is that stress might awaken or aggravate dormant health problems, depending on the degree of internal integrity or vulnerability of the immune system. Most Americans are "stressed" for a multitude of reasons—challenging relationship, demanding job, overdue bills, or poor health—but how can the degree of stress be measured?

How would you rate your stress level on a scale from 1 to 5? Ask a friend to rate her stress level, and compare both of your answers. Let's say you say 4, and she says 5, but you *know* you have more stress than she does. The scale for measuring stress is too subjective and too difficult to measure accurately.

Does your stress rating of 5 have the same intensity as *my* stress level 5? Is it 5 all day long or just some of the time? Besides, how can anyone tell if stress causes MS? Maybe a bad car accident and terrible infection occurred at the same time. Is it possible MS was caused by a combination of these two events?

Intuitively, we know stress is harmful to human health and may worsen autoimmune diseases, but we may never know scientifically. Studies cannot be based on intuition. Only scientifically valid studies are considered meaningful and can be reviewed for their rightful relevance.

What about magnet therapy?

Shortly after my diagnosis, I met with a bunch of girlfriends for a couple of drinks. A young guy sitting next to me on a bar stool rambled on about his success selling full-body magnet sheets to physicians and chiropractors. He asked why I needed assistance walking into the bar. When I told him I had MS, he excitedly suggested that I try his magnetic forms, saying they had produced great results for relieving MS spasms and stress.

He ran out to his car and within a matter of minutes I was sitting on a magnetic sheet positioned from behind my neck to under my butt and thighs close to my knees. He spoke about the product with such exuberance, he almost convinced me that I would be able to walk home. I stayed on the magnetic surface for almost two hours. As our group was ready to leave, I rose hoping to have a tad more spring in my step. Disappointed, I felt no change of any sort.

Rejected for an MS clinical trial

The Ohio State University MS Clinic was a testing site for a new oral MS drug, fampridine (now on the market under brand name, Amprya), and was enrolling study subjects who met the eligibility criteria. This drug was the first to theoretically increase muscle strength, and I definitely wanted to be part of the study. The way the drug worked was different from other drugs and potentially could improve muscle function.

I called the nurse who was overseeing the study protocol to convey my interest in participating as a subject and to get clarification about its design: whether it was blinded (would the doctor or I know if the drug I was taking was real or a placebo?), the length of time the study ran, and the inclusion criteria.

She mentioned that study subjects would be measured by clocking the time it took to walk twenty-five feet before and after taking the study drug. Therefore, participants were required to be able to walk twenty-five feet to be included in the study. What a letdown. I was sitting in a wheelchair, with all the time in the world to participate in a drug study, but I *couldn't walk*! I desperately wanted to try this medication and find out whether it would have even the slightest effect on any muscular function. I would never know, however, because I was rejected from the list of possible study candidates.

When I shared the disheartening news with those who knew of my interest in trying this novel substance, they, too, found it difficult to believe I was rejected. "You want to be in this study *because you can't walk,* and they don't want you in the study *because you can't walk.* You need to be able to walk to be included in the study of a drug that might help you walk?"

Being disqualified from this research project was frustrating, but I understood that the study outcome had to be measurable. Because I couldn't walk, there was no other parameter that could be assessed to evaluate the drug's impact.

Newspaper headline: "Lightning Strikes Woman in Bathtub; MS Gone!"

My sister once told me about a woman with MS who experienced a powerful shock while she was taking a bath. Lightning had struck the metal outside her home, traveled through the bathroom plumbing, penetrated the water, and "reset" her body's electrical system. Her MS symptoms disappeared; she could walk and no longer needed her wheelchair.

The implication: a lightning shock can cure MS.

If nine out of ten MS patients have relapsing-remitting MS, there is a 90 percent chance this woman had it as well. It is possible that she was going into a remission (the natural process of "recovering" from her last MS relapse) about the same time that lightning struck.

Another reason I think this woman had RRMS, not PPMS, is that she was able to immerse herself into water in a bathtub. How the heck did she manage to get herself into a bathtub? I, too, am in a wheelchair but have full-body paralysis. I couldn't get my body into a bathtub on my best day. Even a caregiver wouldn't be able to lift my dead weight over the edge of the tub.

The "lightning-shock-that-cured-MS" scenario is another example of anecdotal "proof." The result may be real, but it does not logically lead to this particular conclusion. In other words, lightning did strike while the woman with MS was taking a bath, and perhaps her symptoms went away. But it would be faulty logic or a hasty generalization to conclude that a lightning shock will cure MS. I'm sure many of us would like to see this studied, but I doubt that many people would line up to be a research candidate for a study that requires enduring lightning-intensity voltage while sitting in bath water.

Anything in print is often interpreted as factual. Think again. A gazillion jokers are out there waiting to see whether their stupid claim on the Internet "goes viral" as the truth.

Can acupuncture treat MS?

A nurse friend of mine knew a young man who was studying homeopathic medicine and acupuncture. Because this person was coming into town, my friend made an appointment for me to visit with him for an acupuncture consultation.

The nurse suggested I pay him at least $50 (in 2000) for the consultation. I questioned this amount because I thought that price for a mere consultation by a student was rather high. Defensively, she blurted out, "I would think that $50 would be nothing if he cured your MS!"

I never had acupuncture from this young man nor anyone else, but this doesn't mean I don't believe acupuncture has healing powers.

I simply don't believe that acupuncture alone is going to cure me from an aggressive case of MS.

The Swank MS diet

Making modifications to one's diet for a therapeutic effect might be a great way to eliminate the need for costly medication. People make changes to what they eat in order to lose weight and control allergies, so why not make an attempt to starve away illnesses?

The diet to improve MS was developed by Dr. Roy Swank. His main focus was on restricting saturated fat consumption to less than ten grams per day and concentrating more on the use of polyunsaturated fats. The diet restrictions sounded safe and healthy, so I gave it a try. I have found no information to support that MS is the result of a nutritional deficiency, but I was open to the dietary change, since I had nothing to lose and everything to gain. I definitely noticed that my weight decreased quickly, but unfortunately, I never saw any improvement in my symptoms.

To ensure that I am giving my body everything it needs, I supplement my diet with the recommended daily allowances of vitamins and minerals with extra emphasis on calcium, vitamin D, vitamin C, and zinc. I have experimented with other nutraceuticals that claim to provide better health for MS patients: lecithin, evening primrose oil, licorice root, DHEA, mega doses of B12 injections, omega-3 fatty acids, and kalawalla. None of these products produced any improvement in my MS symptoms.

The power of positive thinking

A friend encouraged me to relax and de-stress in the earlier stages of my MS to allow my symptoms to improve. I did everything in my power to reduce my stressful thinking and allow my natural ability to "rise above" and restore my physical health. She provided a series of audiotapes instructing me to find my "chakras" and get in touch with my energy fields.

I have always been considered an optimistic person but couldn't figure out why I wasn't positive enough to heal my MS. It took years before I felt confident enough to say I had exercised all the affirmative energy I could muster but am now convinced that all the positive thinking in the world is not going to make me walk again.

What about the power of God?

People wonder if I ever asked God to get rid of my MS. The answer is a resounding, "No." I do, however, pray for strength to *deal* with the disease. Even when you think you are not strong enough to handle greater demands, I believe God knows you are more capable than you may believe.

Conceding the facts

I've tried a host of interventions, both traditional and alternative, including medicinals, supplements, and holistic methods. Some I have either forgotten about or am too embarrassed to mention. All produced disappointing results.

During the first few years following my diagnosis, I closely monitored and scrutinized the MS research landscape. Promises of a cure in five to ten years kept me riveted. I patiently sat at my computer for hours each day searching for information about the latest developments or new advances in MS treatments. I carefully researched and read many news journals, periodicals, and online updates.

After fourteen years and no significant changes in MS therapy, I have conceded that research into a disease moves at a painfully slow pace. Even if it takes a few extra days to come to my attention, I am not as vigilant in my MS research as I used to be. I changed my game plan from looking for the first word of a cure to adapting to and making the best of my life's new status quo.

Even though I've turned my focus away from waiting for a cure to making life with MS more workable, I still keep my ear to the ground and read what's happening in the MS field. I filter out the sounds of gobbledygook and let in the information that seems to matter. The sad part is, little has changed in the fourteen years since I was first diagnosed with MS.

Out of obligation for the betterment of MS research, I contribute information about my ongoing treatment and functional changes to the North American Research Committee on Multiple Sclerosis (http://narcoms.org/) every six months. The website I visit most often is the Myelin Repair Foundation (www.myelinrepair.org/), an organization developed in the early 2000s by a former CEO of a Silicon Valley company who has MS. Being familiar with the slow-moving drug-development process, I am intrigued and inspired by his collaborative research efforts that unite the brainpower of some of the country's largest centers for MS intelligence and encourage acceleration of medical research for myelin repair. Another website I find straightforward, factual, and compassionate is www.acceleratedcure.org.

The topic of MS has gained notoriety, and scores of honorable individuals are now investing their time to increase awareness; raise money; research the causes and cure of MS; or manage the numerous physical, emotional, and social problems associated with the disease. I will continue to await new treatments that may improve my function. In the meantime, I will live my life as fully as I can.

Chapter 4
MS Misconceptions: Appearances Can Be Deceiving

I tried hard to avoid using assistive walking devices like a cane or a wheelchair, stalling the inevitable for as long as possible. Plenty of old people could stand up on their own feet without them—why not me? I attempted to walk unassisted for months after my diagnosis, preferring to lean against walls and other people than use any "handicap" aid.

Remaining self-reliant made me a danger to myself. I often dragged one foot over loose carpet, a threshold, or a slight elevation in the flooring and, consequently, ended up tripping or falling.

I walked unsteadily, and because I used no obvious assistive devices, people often stared at me. After my diagnosis, my tendency to fall confirmed that my body was slowly falling apart. As I began to lose my ability to walk and my confidence, I was bowled over by the reality of my physical deterioration. In this early stage of my progressive MS, I began to feel, "I can't win for losing."

Picking up my daughter from preschool

Before I began using an assistive walking device, symptoms from my MS were the source of many misunderstandings. Here's a good example.

In 1999, I had just picked up my six-year-old daughter from her early childhood school and secured her tightly in a car seat strapped in the backseat of my Lexus sedan. As was my custom, I wrapped a seat belt across her shoulder, then another one over mine when I finally plopped into the driver's seat. Traffic was thin but moving sluggishly on the residential streets of Upper Arlington that day. As I slowly approached a red light at the next intersection, in my rearview mirror, I spotted not one but two city police vehicles driving behind me. I continued driving cautiously for the next several hundred yards. I put on my left turn signal to prepare to slowly move over into the left lane. The police officers driving behind me followed suit.

As I approached the traffic light to turn, I started feeling a bit anxious. I briefly took my eyes off the road and examined my seat belt. Check. I gazed in the rearview mirror to make certain Sophia's was on correctly, too. Check. I turned my car onto my street and continued driving gingerly into our driveway several houses down. The two police cars immediately pulled up against the curb directly in front of our house and activated their obnoxiously bright red and blue rotor lights on top of the cars.

I opened my car door and climbed out, then opened the back door for Sophia and unsnapped her belt buckle to let her out. Then, I stood up straight, rotating my body to look at the men, and leaned against the car.

"Okay. What did I do?" I sincerely wanted to know.

I had asked the question with a strong voice and a smile. They walked across the grassy margin near the curb. As cops do, they appeared to be looking to kick my ass for something I did wrong.

The policeman who was obviously in charge spoke while his partner followed behind. "Ma'am, we just got a call from a concerned mother who watched you walk as you picked up your daughter from Burbank Early Childhood School. She suspected you were intoxicated."

Thank God it wasn't my driving, I thought, and responded to his accusation with relief, knowing it wasn't some traffic violation. "Oh! I have MS."

I quickly thought back to about twenty minutes earlier and how I might have appeared while walking into Burbank. I'm sure I used all the available walls to navigate the hallways. To the typical person who knew nothing of my battle with MS and balance, it must have appeared that I had just kicked back a few. So many thoughts and visuals rushed through my head. It seemed a half hour passed, but it was only a minute or two.

The officer who had originally fixed his eyes on me and suspiciously judged my facial and body movements replied quickly. "Oh, we are so sorry!" he said as he lowered his head and walked backward to his car. I sensed his embarrassment and actually felt sorry for both of them.

I stopped and wondered why they believed me. Why did they readily accept my "alibi" without any credentials or references? Did I *look* like I had MS? What does a person with MS look like, anyway? The truth was, I didn't feel good about their assumption of my innocence, either.

As they were just about to enter their cars, I snapped, "I can show you my handicap placard if you'd like." I leaned against the driver's side door of my car. What was I thinking? It's not like the disability placard is an ID card. Besides, it still doesn't prove I'm an MS club member.

They brushed off the offer to see my placard; but, before I let them disappear into their vehicles, I curiously asked, "Do you know who placed the call to you?"

"Yes, ma'am, we do," they admitted with apologetic voices.

"I really don't care to know who called, but I would appreciate it if you could let her know about my MS. I'm not angry. I could have made the same mistake."

Erroneous airline profiling?

Shortly after my diagnosis in early March 1999, I was returning home from my last scheduled business trip to a new company client in Mobile, Alabama. A last-minute mechanical problem caused the Northwest Airlines flight to be canceled, and I needed to catch an afternoon connecting flight in Detroit.

On the connecting jet headed for Columbus, Ohio, I walked through the long fuselage to my seat, which was almost twenty rows from the front of the plane. Once I got there, I tucked my overnight bag in the luggage storage area above and set my computer bag on the floor under my seat. After I squared away all of my belongings prior to take off, I exited my seat and moved about eight more rows to the bathroom at the back of the plane.

I had thought I would not start my monthly period until I was back home. I was aghast because I started early and was unprepared. I was wearing a sharp-looking New York Jones pantsuit and wanted to check for any "leakage."

I addressed the situation, determined I had a few small spots on my pants, and managed to reassemble myself in the restrictive quarters of the airplane bathroom. I left the small bathroom and plotted a course back to my seat.

Within a minute of sitting down, an attractive, blond flight attendant stood closely above me and said, "Ms. Wolf?" I quickly picked up my head, made full eye contact, and smiled to acknowledge the name belonged to me.

"Could you please walk to the front of the plane?" she asked like a schoolteacher.

All of a sudden, I felt self-conscious and thought others would notice the blood spots on my pants. So, out of sheer embarrassment, I assumed she was referring to my pants and wanted to make certain I was aware of the spot.

"Oh, if this is about the spot on my pants, I already know about it," I whispered with my head lowered behind the seat in front of me.

She gave me a puzzled look and cocked her head to the side. "No." She hesitated while thinking of a way to correct my assumption. I am certain she didn't even know what I was talking about. "The male flight attendant at the front of the plane suspects you're intoxicated."

I quickly processed her words and realized the scenario was no different from what had occurred only a couple of weeks earlier with the Arlington police. "Oh, I have MS." I bravely shook my head, smiled, and quickly pulled out my handicap placard from my purse. I wasn't going to miss the opportunity to show the card this time and waved it a couple of feet above my lap.

"Oh. OK," she responded without a smile or even an apology. She turned around and walked toward the front of the plane.

I sat there imagining how I must have looked from behind walking to my seat and to the bathroom. Yes, I know; I must have walked like I was drunk. This was a big plane with probably more than one hundred seats and fewer than twenty passengers.

I began to realize how wrong and tasteless the attendants' accusation and request were. Demand that I walk to the front of the plane? Why? I wasn't a raucous passenger interrupting others. The person sitting closest to me was at least four rows away. What really angered me was Northwest Airlines had served me alcohol over my "limit" on several previous occasions when I had flown as a first-class passenger. The hypocrisy! Even if I were drunk, who cares? *I wasn't flying the plane!*

I became very sad. So many oppressive thoughts ran through my mind.

So, is this how it's always going to be? I wanted to walk tall and with good posture. Now I felt embarrassed and wondered how I could prevent people from ever again thinking I was drunk. That's when I realized that life as I knew it had come to an end. My eyes began to fill with tears. I kept them shut until we landed on the tarmac in Columbus.

Once the short flight ended, I picked up my shoulder bag from the floor and wheeled my overnight bag with my computer strapped to it down the aisle behind me. At the front of the plane, flight attendants were standing in line at attention with smiles on their faces saying their customary thank-yous and good-byes to exiting passengers.

I was the last person, crawling out from under my rock of shame. As I walked past, each attendant awkwardly turned around to avoid facing me. Even the pilot, who had emerged from the cockpit to bid adieu, deliberately went back into the flight control center as I approached.

Every time I shared my story, friends strongly suggested I press charges against Northwest Airlines, but I couldn't think of a reasonable remedy to request for this "wrongdoing." Only my feelings were hurt and my ego damaged. Maybe an apology? An admission of error?

Soon after this incident, a TV exposé on poor airline service aired. Who do you think was on the top of the "poor service" list? Northwest Airlines. I visualized the probable location of my complaint letter: somewhere three feet down from the top of the stack. Needless to say, I lost my incentive to fight, but I grew from this incident and decided to pick more meaningful disability battles in the future.

You'd think a hospital would know better

I sat in my electric wheelchair in a hospital patient room waiting for a procedure to alleviate my trigeminal neuralgia—the cause of stabbing pain in my face. The admitting nurse asked me kindly if I could move my body onto the bed.

Really? This mischaracterization of my physical abilities while I was in a wheelchair wasn't the first time, nor is it limited to this incident. Frequently, when I meet new people they assume I am able to shake hands or grasp something they hand me. It's flattering that I give an impression of sufficient vibrancy to move my body. But it is also frustrating to think that I need a ventilation tube dangling from my neck to make people understand I am not able to put my arms or legs in motion.

But you look so good!

The stories above exemplify the common misconception that a person with a neurological disability is intoxicated. On the flip side, some people judge a person with reasonably good looks as healthy. This reminds me of the Lorenzo Lammas parody performed by Billy Crystal in the 1980s on *Saturday Night Live*. "Dahling, you look mahvelous! You know, dahling; it is better to *look* good than to *feel* good."

As nice as it might seem to be told you look great even when you feel like crap, it can feel patronizing to the disabled person. It seems as if the person doling out the "compliment" doesn't recognize the disabled person's misery. I'm not saying one should shower a disabled person with such comments as, "I know how you must feel," because sugar-coated pity is equally patronizing. The best approach is to ask open-ended questions, listen, and allow the disabled person to share his or her own feelings. It is important to recognize that a person with a disability has fought some fierce battles, and it would be unconscionable to discredit her emotions or experiences.

What you see is not necessarily what you get

Some people abuse and disrespect the handicap placard for their own selfish purposes. They take a spot reserved for the handicapped because other parking places are difficult to find, in an inconvenient location, or far from the front door.

Handicap parking spaces are for people who have trouble walking. The plastic, royal-blue-and-white card hooked on the rearview mirror affords people with disabilities the privilege of parking closer to their destinations in public parking spaces. Handicap placard "vigilantes" have minimized improper use by policing the "medically necessary" need for the shortened walk. On the flipside, be careful whom you criticize for what might appear to be handicap-placard abuse.

Here is another story: I was just diagnosed with MS and used my new handicap placard for parking in front of a large grocery store in Upper Arlington. As I entered the store, I recognized a doctor I had formerly worked with at a local nursing home, and I called out to him as he was examining vegetables. "Hello, Dr. Jones" (not his real name).

He was holding a green pepper and immediately looked at me with a sour face and said, "You know, people with handicap placard's typically can't walk."

I thought he was pulling my leg, hoping that I would laugh. When I realized he didn't remember me, nor was he joking, I quickly replied, "Hi, Dr. Jones, it's me, Lauri Epitropoulos [I used the name he knew me by]. I was just diagnosed with MS."

"Well, I'm doing a little investigative work because my sister-in-law just became handicapped and can never find a handicap parking space because so many people who are *not* handicapped take up all these spaces," he replied curtly, without an apology for assuming I was an abuser.

Hit me in the head, why don't you?

My personal experience reminded me of a blog for MS patients who complained about non-handicapped people using the reserved parking spaces.

This story describes an incident about a man and his wife, both with MS. The man used a wheelchair, and his wife used a cane. One afternoon, they waited patiently for a handicap space to open, intending to grab it before anyone else did. They were foiled by a pretty blonde in a shiny yellow sports car who had been waiting for the same parking space. The man and his wife were disappointed, but, only moments later, another parking space a couple slots away from the yellow sports car became available. They quickly parked before it, too, was taken.

The man with MS assembled his wheelchair after he pulled it out from the backseat of their sedan and snapped at the woman who was exiting the sports car, "Hey, what gives you the right to use that handicap placard?"

The woman was noticeably irritated and clung to a shopping cart with both fists clenched. She leaned as she walked, grabbed at her calf, pulled off a prosthetic leg, and threw it forcefully over her shoulder, attempting to hit the man.

That story might have been crafted to get your attention. It certainly got mine. Perhaps it wasn't entirely accurate, but the point is that many of the reasons people require a "handicap" designation aren't visible to onlookers. A valid placard requires an order from a licensed physician. Those unable to produce a placard when they are confronted are fined, and these fees have increased two and a half times in the past several years. Disability laws are rightfully carrying greater weight than ever.

Chapter 5
Juggling Multiple Health Problems with Multiple Sclerosis

W e have virtually no control over the ravages of MS itself; so, in addition to controlling inflammation of nerve tissue and "relapses," we also have to pay attention to the myriad complications brought on by the disease. Treatment for consequential complications of MS, such as spasticity, incontinence, and fatigue, are pivotal to managing this disease; but other non-MS health issues are just as likely to occur in MS patients as with the general population.

The loss of physical functioning in MS can be a distraction from other potential health problems that may be lurking. You should undertake preventive measures to ensure your health and monitor for disease indicators, including high blood sugar, cholesterol, blood pressure, and pulse.

Fundamental treatment of MS

The theory behind MS, at least RRMS, is that the body's immune system is in overdrive and attacks its own neurological system. This attack (relapse, exacerbation, or flare) results in defilement of the myelin tissue surrounding the nerves. The inflammatory damage to this outer layer of the nerve interrupts the conduction of electrical energy, which is necessary for controlling various muscular and bodily functions.

MS treatments are designed to subdue the immune system and minimize the number of these relapses, which may lead to secondary-progressive MS. PPMS, on the other hand, destroys nerve function from the get-go and never takes a break. In addition, it is unresponsive to immunosuppressive drugs, and there are no FDA-approved medications to tame the wiles of this beast or repair the injury it leaves behind. Like most medications, those used to control MS relapses have uninvited side effects.

Since my subtype of MS was unclear at the time of my diagnosis, I was initially treated for RRMS with a series of immunosuppressive drugs: Copaxone (glatirimer), a daily self-administered subcutaneous shot; Avonex (beta interferon), a weekly intramuscular injection; Novantrone (mitoxantrone), a chemotherapeutic agent infused intravenously as an aggressive attempt to halt my MS progression; Solu-Medrol (methylprednisolone), a one-time run with the cortisone intravenous infusion; and methotrexate oral tablets, a drug also used to treat other diseases, including cancer.

When I was first diagnosed with "probable MS," my neurologist and I agreed on Copaxone. The National MS Society clearly recommended that all newly diagnosed MS patients begin immunosuppressive therapy promptly. Although my subtype of MS was unknown before January 1999, having this specific information was not as much a priority as it is today. Consequently, I was treated as if I had RRMS.

I questioned my neurologist about whether he thought it was worthwhile to use any of these immunosuppressive medications if I had PPMS and not RRMS. He believed that medications the FDA approved for MS were tested on the RRMS subtype simply because the number of relapses occurring with or without the drug was "easy to count." In contrast, measuring the impact of a drug intended to *slow the progression* of a disease such as MS is difficult.

We selected Copaxone from the ABC (Avonex, Betaseron, Copaxone, and now Rebif) injectable drug choices because of its combination of high efficacy and low incidence of side effects. Although daily subcutaneous injections were required, the skin didn't need to be pierced any deeper than for an insulin shot. This was less risky than shots given deeper into the muscle tissue.

I needed to select and rotate six different injection sites within a seven-day period for my Copaxone injections. My overall encounter with this drug was favorable, but an unusual skin reaction occurred on two occasions. Scattered on both the left and right sides of my abdomen, back, upper butt, and upper arms were red, raised patches revealing a historic mapping of every shot I ever received at all six different injection sites.

I took Copaxone for two years, but since my physical functioning continued to deteriorate at the same pace, my neurologist decided to try a different immunosuppressive drug and switched me to Avonex.

Although I followed the tutorial on self-administering this drug, I wimped out and relied on a friend, who was a nurse, to give it to me in my butt each week. The decreased frequency was welcome, but the post-dose washed-out feeling the next day was not. I needed to include this downtime in my work and social planning every week. This "dragged-down" side effect and lack of any noticeable improvement led to my decision to stop using Avonex after more than one year.

My neurologist then tried a three-day course of IV methylprednisolone to halt any muscular deterioration and possibly improve my ability to walk. A nurse visited my home to set up the daily IV infusions. Even this short run of steroid injections left me feeling beat up and gave me insomnia. I practiced good "sleep hygiene," meaning I only slept in my bed without watching TV or reading books, but I absolutely could not close my eyelids. A warm glass of milk was worthless. I finally took a tablet of Ambien (zolpidem), a sedative-hypnotic drug prescribed for sleep. It worked, and I slumbered hard and fast.

IV Novantrone (mitoxantrone) is an injectable chemotherapeutic drug originally approved for certain leukemias, lymphomas, and metastatic breast and prostate cancers. This drug later received FDA approval for SPMS. The indigo-ink-colored liquid is prescribed for infusion intravenously every three months. Since Novantrone can damage the heart muscle, an electrocardiogram (EKG) must be performed prior to receiving each quarterly dose to determine whether the heart appears healthy enough to start or endure continued therapy.

Nausea is common with Novantrone, as with most chemotherapeutic drugs; so doctors frequently preemptively prescribe antinausea drugs to be taken beforehand. I received a prescription of oral Kytril (ondansetron), which was very effective in keeping me from feeling nauseated.

Another side effect of Novantrone is hair loss (alopecia), which can occur in one-third of those using the drug. The hair loss side effect cannot be prevented. Hair loss may seem to be merely cosmetic or superficial, but I'm certain the dramatic change in my appearance affected me emotionally. I didn't feel good about the way it changed my looks. According to my hairdresser, I lost about 60 percent of my hair within a month after my first and only dose. Additionally and unexpectedly, when my hair did grow back, the texture changed from straight and smooth to frizzy and curly.

Methotrexate (MTX), an oral chemotherapeutic agent, is used for psoriasis and approved for secondary-progressive MS. MTX was prescribed for me because the other drugs were not slowing my deterioration. I took this drug along with the customary addition of folic acid for almost two years; it produced no useful improvement in my MS.

After numerous attempts to halt my declining MS condition with immunomodulating drugs, I continued to progress on an even-paced downward slope that never changed from the time I first remember having MS symptoms. Attempts to interrupt its path of destruction were futile. I was convinced I had PPMS instead of RRMS and stopped making additional efforts to change the course of the disease.

Common health problems with MS

Regardless of subtype, all people with MS are subject to the same assortment of additional health problems and, consequently, treatment options. Symptom management is the name of the game in MS. Sometimes, the only treatment is simply to control any nuisance problems brought on by the disease. Many of these problems are discussed in-depth later in the book.

• Incontinence: Bladder leaking without a cough, chuckle, or sneeze!
Incontinence is difficult to treat because the medications prescribed have anticholinergic side effects that make your brain foggy, your mouth and eyes dry, and your bowels slow to move. Incontinence is hardest to manage when urinary retention is also a problem. You want to turn off the leaky bladder but not so much that you can't pee at all. Most medications for urinary problems are to control either incontinence or urinary retention but not both. I will discuss more about bladder control in Chapter 6, "When the Levee Breaks: Loss of Bladder Control."

• Spasticity: Crazy, tight, and sometimes painful muscle contractions
Spasticity has been the longest-running health issue with my MS; its severity continues to evolve. I will discuss the subject of spasticity more thoroughly in Chapter 7, "Battle Between Brain and Brawn: Spasticity."

• Peripheral neuropathy: Burning or itching in the limbs
I had driven to the Cleveland Clinic with a colleague to meet with a neurologist at the MS Center for another opinion on my MS treatment. I was disappointed and walked away feeling hopeless, as even an astute physician from the world-renowned Cleveland Clinic had no secret MS cures and couldn't fix me. She did, however, order gabapentin for my burning, itchy feet, a classic sign of peripheral neuropathy. She spurned the notion that my MS subtype was most likely primary progressive.

• Depression: More than just "the blues"
Almost 50 percent of MS patients suffer with depression.[1] Depression in MS is treated with antidepressant medication, often for a lifetime, with or without psychotherapy. The doctor may conduct tests to assess

---

1 Goldman Consensus Group, "The Goldman Consensus Statement on Depression in Multiple Sclerosis," *Multiple Sclerosis* 11 (2005): 328–37.

whether antidepressant therapy is warranted and effective initially or over the long term.

The different kinds of antidepressants are categorized by the neurotransmitter they most notably increase: serotonin, norepinephrine, or dopamine. One or more antidepressants may be selected based on which neurochemical level they enhance and the side effects each has.

The SSRIs, or selective serotonin reuptake inhibitors, include names such as Zoloft (sertraline), Prozac (fluoxetine), Paxil (paroxetine), and Lexapro (escitalopram). Antidepressants such as Effexor (venlafaxine) and Cymbalta (duloxetine) work to increase a combination of norepinephrine and serotonin.

I've tried Zoloft, Paxil, Effexor, and Cymbalta for one reason or another; and each made me feel "spacey"—like I was walking through a cloud. Since these medications increased serotonin, I decided to stay with one that didn't elevate this neurochemical.

Wellbutrin (bupropion) tends to increase dopamine but not serotonin. This drug is considered an "activating" antidepressant, less likely to cause sexual side effects and more likely to cause insomnia and precipitate anxiety.

Before I was diagnosed with MS, I saw my internist about the weird physical symptoms I was having. Because I was recently remarried, employed full-time, and feeling stressed out, my physician prescribed antidepressant therapy because he suspected my lack of balance and muscle weakness might be manifestations of depression.

My preference was bupropion, which had two potential additional benefits: aiding in smoking cessation and improving adult attention deficit disorder (ADD). Bupropion has successfully lifted my mood for more than fourteen years with no notable side effects. On the other hand, it has never curbed my desire for a cigarette (although smoking is more likely behavioral rather than a nicotine dependency with me). I have never been diagnosed with ADD, but I have noticed my thought processes have become noticeably clearer and more organized since I have been taking this medication.

Most would argue the combination of antidepressant therapy and psychotherapy produces the best results for dealing with depression. During the first year after my MS diagnosis, I visited with a psychologist to help me accept my new disabling health situation with greater confidence. I don't know if this helped, but I'm certain it didn't hurt.

In general, all antidepressants are considered to have equal therapeutic success, and their side-effect profiles are their only real differences. Therefore, an antidepressant is typically selected based on its side-effect profile as clinicians try to base their selection on the one that has the "best" side effects for the patient. In other words, doctors choose an antidepressant with the side effects they think a patient can best tolerate.

• *Anxiety: What, me worry?*
People with MS frequently experience anxiety. Some antidepressants are also prescribed to treat anxiety. For example, Paxil (paroxetine) is approved for symptoms of anxiety or jitteriness.

When I was first diagnosed with MS, my neurologist prescribed Inderal (propranolol), a beta-blocker, which controlled the excessive beating of my heart that would occur whenever I became extremely nervous. Like a domino effect, my pounding chest would bring on an anxiety spell. I took only a couple of tablets of this medication, but nearly ten years later when I wanted to replace the expired tablets, my doctor explained he no longer prescribed the "cardiac medication" for this purpose. I was disappointed because the product had worked well for my anxiety.

Since bupropion can instigate anxiety, my family practitioner decided to reduce this medication from 150 mg SR (sustained release) twice daily to once daily. Lowering the dose did not decrease my anxiety level, unfortunately. In addition, after four months on the lower dose, my depression worsened, and I needed to return to my original twice-daily dosage.

The most effective anti-anxiety medication I have used is Ativan (lorazepam). I did not experience any residual sedation or "hangover" effect. Also, when I was suffering from pain of trigeminal neuralgia (see Chapter 9), I was given IV Ativan while I was in the hospital. This Valium-like drug effectively subdued my emotional state along with the severe muscle tension in my face, neck, and shoulders and tamed my hypervigilance in anticipation of pain "fits." (Although I favor this medicine, benzodiazepines such as lorazepam, should be used on a very limited basis only, as they can lead to drug dependence.)

• Fatigue: Feeling "wasted," "fried," or "burned out"

Fatigue refers to a state of mental exhaustion, overwhelming physical weakness, and lack of motivation. Although some amount of fatigue is common for anyone with a busy adult life, with or without kids, it can be greatly exacerbated by a neurological disorder like MS. A couple of pharmaceutical options exist that should be discussed with a doctor.

Symmetrel (amantadine) is a dopamine activator commonly used as an antiviral medication against certain strains of flu and in the treatment of Parkinson's disease; it is also used to treat fatigue. The typical dose is 100 mg once or twice daily. Symmetrel was the first medication I received for fatigue. Not only did it fail to combat my fatigue, sadly, it even caused me to feel slightly sedated. My neurologist discontinued this medicine and ordered Ritalin (methylphenidate) instead.

Ritalin is a stimulant, controlled substance typically used for attention deficit hyperactivity disorder (ADHD). When I took it I felt edgy, anxious, and overstimulated. My heart beat so fast and hard I was sure it would escape my chest. This medication generated too much excitability even after I lowered my dosage, so I stopped taking it. After several years, my neurologist said that, like most prescribers, he no longer prescribed Ritalin for fatigue.

For a little pep that can't be supplied by a cup of coffee, I'll grab my "MS upper"—Nuvigil (armodafinil)—the isomer or "fraternal twin" of Provigil (modafinil), a drug that was originally approved by the FDA for narcolepsy and to "improve wakefulness" in third-shift workers.

Unfortunately, my insurance company won't approve Nuvigil for MS fatigue even though its use for this condition has been extensively published in medical journals. Nuvigil is expensive, so ask for as many samples as you can get your hands on.

To increase my wakefulness, I typically take a half of a 150 mg Nuvigil on an as-needed basis. I seem to have the "plateau" effect with Nuvigil, which means I don't achieve a greater amount of energy with 150 mg than I do with 75 mg.

Nuvigil has not been able to convert a sleepy day into one full of energy, but it can modestly improve my degree of vitality. For instance, if fatigue is measured on a scale from 1 to 10 (with 10 being the worst), Nuvigil might reduce my fatigue level from a score of 8 to a score of 5. This medication can reduce my tiredness but cannot perform spectacular turnarounds.

Caffeine puts a little fire in my engine, as it does for millions of Americans, as evidenced by the popularity and success of Starbucks. Although the pendulum swings back and forth with new medical information, it seems the latest research on caffeine is solidly favorable.[2] As with any food or medicine, caffeine should be used in moderation. Some physicians tell their patients not to ingest it if they have breast cancer. Consult with a physician regarding caffeine use.

• *Heat: The great MS offender*
My motto: "Heat is my kryptonite." I have found that avoiding spending time in the heat is best for me, as it can overtake any effort to improve muscle strength and fatigue. Temperatures higher than 80° F begin to slow me down considerably. Of course, high temperatures are exacerbated when the air is moist, so I turn off my home humidifier in the summer. My body is sensitive to temperature changes, and I can detect a paltry one- to two-degree difference in my indoor environment.

Exposure to the sun in small doses is healthy because it converts an inactive form of vitamin D into an active one in the skin. Vitamin D

---

2 "NIH Study Finds That Coffee Drinkers Have Lower Risk of Death," *NIH News*, May 16, 2012; http://www.nih.gov/news/health/may2012/nci-16.htm.

is a necessary vehicle for the absorption of calcium. Only ten minutes of UVB sunlight can provide up to 10,000 IU vitamin D conversion.[3] However, I try to avoid the intoxicating exposure to sun for long periods of time. This can be difficult as I am easily mesmerized by its warmth.

Ceiling fans run continuously in my house. I also wear a "cooling vest" prefilled with a substance that can be tossed into the freezer and pulled out to use on a very hot day. I bought an inexpensive vest through Amazon Marketplace for those days when my daughter plays softball and I expect to be outdoors in the heat for a few hours. Also, I am equipped with a small spray pump filled with water to cool my body.

Alternatively, I have a handy battery-operated fan that can be worn around my neck. I carry a washcloth in a container filled with cold water, ready to ring out and cool down hot, sweaty skin on my temples, back of the neck, and wrists. I also keep a bottle of drinking water available to stay hydrated and make my kidneys happy.

• *Constipation: How to get things moving*
Constipation is a common problem for many but especially for MS patients and others with decreased mobility. Just as MS damages the ability to operate muscles in arms and legs, the same slowdown occurs within the intestinal walls.

The best treatment for constipation is prevention. The most fundamental aspects of prevention include drinking plenty of fluids and consuming adequate amounts of fiber-containing foods. The foods I have found best for fiber and bulk are broccoli, popcorn, and apples.

The recommended fiber amount is 20 to 35 grams and water is eight eight-ounce glasses each day. Physical movement is very beneficial; so for immobilized patients, prevention techniques are important. With no muscle movement in the intestines the amount

---

3 D. Kotz, "Time in the Sun: How Much Is Needed for Vitamin D?," *US News/Health*, June 23, 2008.

of fiber consumed may be worthless and a stimulant laxative might be necessary.

I have tried all therapeutic options for constipation including stool softeners, bowel stimulants, osmotic agents, suppositories, and enemas. Stool softeners such as Colace (docusate sodium) soften hard stool to make it easier to pass. I've never found Colace helpful since the muscles in my intestinal wall are not active. A better effect usually occurs when used in combination with a laxative like senna, as in Pericolace. Bowel irritants such as senna and Dulcolax (bisacodyl) move contents through the "lazy" lumen of the gut. Laxatives seem to work best when taken the day before you expect to produce a bowel movement.

Osmotic agents such as Miralax (polyethylene glycol) and lactulose draw water from the intestinal walls to help soften bowel contents, making for easier movement. I have found polyethylene glycol powder in water pleasant as it is tasteless and effective after two to three days. A glycerin suppository can also be inserted rectally to irritate the lining of the lower colon to help empty its contents.

For more severe cases of constipation, a saline/phosphorus enema might be used. Rectal enemas are best administered while lying down. After administration, wait ten to fifteen minutes before returning to the toilet.

All of these products are good depending on the severity of constipation. I must consume an adequate amount of fiber-containing foods as a basis for good bowel health. Stool softeners on their own are not as effective as those with a stimulant laxative like senna. If no bowel movement occurs for four to five days, I use a glycerin suppository; if that's ineffective, I turn to Miralax at bedtime. I rarely use a saline enema unless all other solutions fail.

I have also tried a novel drug for constipation called Amitiza (lubiprostone). The pharmacologic effect increases the motility of the muscles in the intestines (peristalsis) to help eliminate its contents. Amitiza is available in 24 mcg and 8 mcg tablets. Although the 24 mcg tablets were very effective, they gave me stomach cramps, so I tried the lower-dose tablets twice each day. However, 8 mcg tablets were not very effective and still produced stomach cramps. I stopped using Amitiza.

• *Vision problems with MS*

Vision problems are common in MS. I was diagnosed with Uhthoff's syndrome by my ophthalmologist after I experienced blurred vision in one eye when I exercised. Double vision (diplopia) in my peripheral fields and jerking eye movements (nystagmus) occurred later, especially when I was concentrating on a stationary object.

Double vision in my peripheral fields interfered with safe driving. My side views were distorted when I turned my head. This was mostly a problem when I needed to check my left-side blind spot before making a left turn. I learned to use my rearview mirrors frequently before moving my vehicle.

One unexpected vision problem arose when I decided to purchase bifocals after a recent eye exam. I needed two strengths, and I knew I would not be able to interchange two different spectacles without assistance. I opted for "transitional" bifocal lenses, which are more fashion friendly, as they have invisible lines of demarcation between the bottom part for reading and the top for seeing things in the distance.

When my eyeglasses arrived, I could not identify the area on the lens for reading. I was convinced the optical center erred on the creation of a true bifocal lens and returned the glasses to the store. After checking the strength of the lenses, the person I talked to reassured me that the glasses were in fact bifocals. In disbelief, I asked her to draw a circle with a felt tip pen to illustrate the area for reading. She circled one area the size of a pencil eraser on each lens.

I chuckled and said, "No wonder! With my MS, I could never keep my eyes still long enough to focus on these little areas!" Apologetically, she said, "Oh, had I known you had MS, I would have never sold you this type of lens. I just worked with an optometrist who warned me not to sell transitional lenses to patients with MS because their eyes move around far too rapidly." She immediately ordered a *traditional* pair of bifocals for me.

• *Pain in my eyes*

About two to three times each year I am struck with a piercing eye pain that seems to originate behind my eyeball. The pain is not well controlled with pressure, so I just keep my eye closed to prevent it from moving around much. Finally, the pain disappears on its own within one to two hours. Ibuprofen 400 mg sometimes softens the severity of the pain.

• *Difficulty breathing*

The diaphragm and other muscles involved in breathing can become weak with MS. Therefore, deep inhalation and exhalation becomes difficult. People with MS may also be unable to clear their lungs by coughing. This is the reason a respiratory infection can have perilous consequences.

After three night trips to the emergency room for breathing treatments, I made an appointment to be evaluated by an allergist. The allergist conducted a routine skin test by applying a sampling of liquid allergens to scratches he deliberately created on the inside of my forearm. After trying several known causes of allergies, such as pollen, grass, and weeds, he applied cat dander; and—*bingo!*—I produced a well-defined raised, red area and was diagnosed with a cat allergy.

The first step to control my allergy was giving my darling kitty a good home at a friend's house. The allergist, however, ordered a home nebulizer unit and wrote a prescription for Pulmicort (budesonide), an inhaled steroid to reduce any inflammation in my lungs, and Xopenex (levalbuterol, like albuterol but with fewer possible heart palpitations), a bronchodilator to help me breathe. Once the cat dander had been eliminated from the fibers of my furniture and clothing, I no longer needed the breathing medications.

Osteoporosis: Them bones, them bones ...

A person who is immobilized, as I am, is at the highest risk for developing osteoporosis. Without weight-bearing exercise, bone tissue dramatically weakens leaving the skeletal infrastructure in danger of breaking more easily. A break resulting in a hip fracture can keep a person in bed for weeks and require nursing-home care. Pressure sores and pulmonary embolism pose another threat.

Adults are encouraged to consume an adequate daily amount of calcium and vitamin D. The recommended amount of calcium is 1,000–1,500 mg each day. A minimal intake of vitamin D is 400 IU, but some literature advises 800 IU daily. Other sources tout even higher doses, and still others recommend that the maximum amount of daily vitamin D not exceed 2,000 IU.

Recently, my physician discovered that my vitamin D level was low despite a steady intake of 800 IU vitamin D each day. With so much emphasis on the benefits of vitamin D supplementation, I began taking chewable Caltrate D three times a day. Each tablet of Caltrate D contains 600 mg calcium with 400 IU vitamin D. The Centrum tablet I take at bedtime also contains 300 mg calcium and 400 IU vitamin D; therefore, my total daily amounts of calcium and vitamin D are 2,100 mg and 1,600 IU, respectively.

Bone mass density testing

A bone mass density (BMD) measurement can determine how tightly compacted bone tissue is compared to "normal." I was diagnosed with osteopenia, meaning my bones were "on their way" to osteoporosis. This faltering BMD level was a wake-up call. Since I wasn't adequately protected from osteoporosis with calcium and vitamin D intake, I suggested to my gynecologist that I begin using a bisphosphonate like Fosamax (alendronate), Actonel (risendronate), or Boniva (ibondronic acid) to prevent the further loss of bone and possibly increase bone density.

Bisphosphonates can be irritating to the esophagus; therefore, if you take one, you should remain sitting upright for at least one half hour to prevent reflux. I needed to take this medication first thing in the morning on an empty stomach with only water (about eight ounces) and no other medications, coffee, or tea that might interfere with its absorption.

I took Boniva, advertised on TV by cute little Sally Field, spokesperson for this product. Boniva is convenient, as I only had to take it once each month. Soon after, I was required to change to a less costly, once-a-week bisphosphonate, Fosamax (alendronate), per my health insurance company.

After nearly three years of diligent bisphosphonate, vitamin D, and calcium use, I was disappointed to learn that my most recent spinal bone mass density landed in the osteoporotic range. Bone tissue cannot be replaced, so I must be careful to prevent falls and subsequent breaks. (This shows how important weight-bearing exercise is to increasing and maintaining bone strength!)

Marijuana for pain

Several states recognize and are decriminalizing the use of marijuana to control pain and spasticity in MS patients. Marijuana is already accepted in some states for recreational and medical uses. To avoid emotional and intellectual instability, I prefer alternatives to a psychogenic drug for the relief of pain and spasticity. I am satisfied with the spasticity relief I get from my baclofen pump but would consider use of marijuana for uncontrollable pain.

Circulation problems from MS

In MS, the nerves don't always deliver messages to the muscles. This inability affects even the tiny muscles within vascular walls and valves of the veins that pump blue, oxygen-deprived blood back to the lungs for reoxygenation. When these valves can't do their job, blood collects in the legs. Poor circulation results in inadequate movement of white blood cells to fight infection. For this reason, the feet of people with MS should be treated like diabetic feet. Toenails should be cut straight across by a podiatrist.

To improve circulation, raise your legs (best at a height above your heart) whenever possible. My physician ordered a twin-sized hospital bed for home. Nine years later, I continue to use this bed and am able to elevate my feet.

The best remedy for reducing swelling, or edema, in my ankles and feet is to elevate them whenever I can. I also take a diuretic (hydrochlorothiazide) every night. Diuretics help eliminate excess water in the skin tissue and increase the need for urination. Although most people take diuretics in the morning so they can use the toilet during the day, I take mine at bedtime because I am catheterized during the night.

To go along with the poor circulation in my feet, my toes are purple. My feet have normal, flesh-tone color after I have been lying down but quickly change to a deep purple as soon as they drop to the floor while I am sitting in my wheelchair.

I am self-conscious about my foot color, and I *always* wear pants—never shorts—to hide my feet and keep from having them examined by onlookers. This shade of purple is alarming to those unaware of my illness. I cover them with sheer stockings 365 days a year to deflect questions like, "Does your doctor know about your feet?" and "Is there anything you can take for that?" Of course, the answers are always yes and no.

When I'm not wearing sheer knee-high "trouser" nylons, I have on support stockings to help push blood back to my heart. Support hose are available in different pressure ranges from 18–20 mm HG to 30–40 mm HG. The higher the "strength" the more difficult they are to put on and can be counterproductive if they produce more constriction, especially in the toes.

Getting rid of "the dreaded monthly period"
I was diagnosed as perimenopausal at forty-seven years old and still have moderate to heavy monthly periods. My hands were weak and fumbled easily, making it difficult to attend to my monthly feminine

hygiene needs. I was immediately sold on the concept of a new pro-gesterone-coated flexible plastic intrauterine device (IUD). The Merina was painlessly inserted into my uterus. Six years later, my periods have not completely stopped, but I only spot lightly about every three or four months.

Treating and preventing non-MS problems

Unfortunately, treating ailments, rather than preventing them, can become the norm. A disease like MS can be a distraction from checking for additional health concerns. Like everyone else, people with MS can become ill as a result of other conditions, such as hypertension, elevated cholesterol, high blood sugar, and overactive or underactive thyroid.

When I had my cholesterol checked, my total cholesterol level was a shocking 268 mg/dL. I was immediately started on Lipitor 10 mg daily. Within six weeks my cholesterol levels had dropped an astounding 54 percent to 136 mg/dL! Lipitor is now available as a generic (atorvastatin), which helps with expense. My liver enzymes are also monitored periodically.

Besides routinely checking blood pressure, cholesterol levels, and blood sugar, here are some examples of other diagnostics that may be performed regularly:

- Mammograms
- Prostate checks
- Colonoscopies (check for colon cancer)
- Eye examinations (for vision, glaucoma, macular degeneration)
- Bone mass density scans

Talk to your healthcare professional about staying current on your immunizations, such as:

- Influenza (annual flu vaccine)
- Tetanus
- Pneumococcal

Optional immunizations to consider include the following:

- Human papillomavirus (HPV)
- Hepatitis A and B
- Meningitis
- Tuberculosis check
- Herpes zoster (shingles)

My MS condition has been complicated by a multitude of health issues. The core of MS revolves around muscle weakness, which cannot be stopped or fixed; but the symptoms of fatigue, depression, constipation, and many others can often be managed successfully.

Chapter 6
When the Levee Breaks: Loss of Bladder Control

L osing control of my bladder has been, hands down, the most profoundly undignified consequence of my MS experience. The adage, "You don't know what you've got till it's gone" can't be better defined than when you can't walk or pull your own pants down to use the bathroom by yourself.

Here we go: The start of my battle with incontinence

My first "accident" happened during an intimate encounter with my then-husband, David. Since I was pregnant, the terribly embarrassing incident was blamed on a weak bladder from hormone changes. After being diagnosed with MS two years later, I realized that the dreadful occurrence was actually a harbinger of a disease soon to manifest itself.

The initial problem I had to tackle, besides balance, was urinary incontinence. Within the first two years of my diagnosis, I complained about it to my neurologist. He wrote a prescription for Ditropan (oxybutynin), a drug to prevent me from leaking urine.

Ditropan was an effective medication for keeping me dry but at the expense of urinary retention. I could hardly pee at all. My neurologist used a portable ultrasound device to measure the amount of residual urine retained after trying to empty my bladder. He determined the volume of urine to be unacceptably high (greater than 200 mL). So my Ditropan was discontinued, and I was instructed to self-catheterize several times each day to assure that my bladder was completely emptied.

Attempting to self-catheterize

A home-care nurse came to my house to teach me how to perform urinary self-catheterization. This procedure is tricky for a woman but especially difficult with unsteady hands and fingers caused by MS.

I tried to hold a mirror still with my clumsy left hand and grasp the short plastic catheter with the weak fingers on my right. Even after numerous tries, it was impossible to find the X on my genital map. The hole for the urethra is incredibly tiny and camouflaged by the surrounding labial skin. Dragging the hard hollow tube over the extremely sensitive genital area was uncomfortable. I grew hot and bothered and decided I just couldn't do the job. I gave up.

If a genie offered me three wishes, one of my wishes would be to empty my bladder and use the toilet the "old-fashioned way," like a normal person.

Seeking a better way to urinate: The urology consult

I failed miserably at self-catheterization, so this method was no longer a treatment option for my mixed incontinence/retention problem.

I consulted with a urologist who presented two choices in early 2000: wear an indwelling Foley catheter around the clock or have a suprapubic catheter surgically placed in my bladder through my lower abdomen.

Both methods were equally unattractive. My risk of urinary tract infections would increase, and each required wearing a urine drain bag, which I found comparable to a prison ball and chain. Also, neither approach would restore my ability to urinate normally. I was determined to find another solution.

Struggling to get on the potty all by myself!

My legs finally gave up, and I began relying on a wheelchair at the start of 2002. The biggest challenge I faced four to six times each day was the effort to go to the bathroom.

I struggled to maneuver my manual wheelchair in the bathroom, clench my hands around the arms of my wheelchair, push my butt straight up off my seat, grip a towel rack—mounted on the wall at shoulder height—to stand, grab hold of the elastic waistband of my pants, pull them down below my butt, pivot, and quickly plop my bare bottom on the toilet seat.

I needed to psych myself into catapulting my body into a standing position—sometimes five or six tries—before I could finally get my pants down and move my naked bottom onto the potty seat. Often, the process took too long, and I lost bladder control. Wet spots on my pants began to be the rule rather than the exception, but bladder-leaking accidents were not the biggest problem I wanted to avoid.

My biggest fear was falling while I was in the bathroom and being unable to get back into my wheelchair. I prayed that either someone would hear me yell or I would be within arm's reach of a phone and someone would answer and get help for me. Despite weighing only about 125 pounds, my tall body was awkward to pick up from the floor and sometimes required two people.

Bulky incontinence pads

The next assault from MS was spontaneously leaking urine for no apparent reason; I didn't cough, laugh, or sneeze. To protect my clothing from these unpredictable "accidents," I wore a heavily advertised incontinence product: Poise pads.

These supposedly absorbent pads weren't as effective as I expected.[1] Pee seemed to run right over the convex surface instead of into its fibers; the pads didn't keep me perfectly dry. Plus, when I went to the bathroom to change a soiled pad, I usually needed to take off my wet underpants and replace them with new, dry ones.

Unlike panty liners or the occasional mini pad, incontinence pads were uncomfortably bulky. They were a constant reminder of humiliation and my doom of always needing them tucked between my legs. Also, on a vain note, thong underwear and incontinence pads had no business being paired.

Depends (the only acceptable "D" word)

My bladder incontinence continued to worsen; and as my condition

---

1 In fairness to the manufacturer of Poise pads, my experience with this product was in the early 2000s. At the time of this writing in 2012, the family of Poise pad choices has increased and perhaps so has the absorbency.

declined, I couldn't get my naked bottom to the toilet fast enough to prevent trickling. So, if I got pee on my pants, I needed to start the arduous process of taking them off and putting on fresh ones.

Dressing was the toughest job I had each day. To appreciate the complicated nature of changing clothes, imagine putting on and taking off a shirt, underwear, pair of pants, socks, and shoes with only one hand. My legs were stiff and would hardly bend at the knee. Sliding a foot into openings of pants was nearly impossible. My fingers couldn't grasp clothing, and a reaching tool to improve my grip didn't help because my hands were too frail.

I even limited my fluid intake to decrease my urine output, but it didn't seem to make much difference. My urethra became a broken, open faucet. I saw the TV ads; I heard the jokes. And now I was fated to wear them: Depends absorbent briefs.

Whenever I thought about purchasing Depends, I would visualize the parody skit on *Saturday Night Live (SNL)* for a product called "Oops, I Sh** My Pants," where an older husband shares with his wife his secret reliance on a disposable brief to protect against incontinence and interruptions to his normal, active lifestyle. The husband in the skit conducts an exaggerated, tasteless representation of mixed bladder and bowel incontinence waste by pouring a half-gallon of gross brown liquid into the brief as a demonstration of its absorbent capacity. There isn't much on *SNL* that doesn't make me laugh, but I found the intended humor difficult to appreciate.

Wearing these unsightly bottoms for the first time was a mortifying experience and one I prayed was only temporary. I never outgrew my deep resentment toward Depends and will eternally reject my need to rely on them.

These disposable pants are called "Depends" in my home to avoid the term adult "diapers," a word I find atrocious and degrading. All my personal-care aides (PCAs) are firmly instructed never to use the "d" word but instead to refer to them by their well-known brand name.

(The only way to truly appreciate the ghastly experience of wearing a pair of Depends is to try wearing one. Then, restrain your bladder until you can't hold your pee any longer, and deny yourself access to a toilet or any place else but the pair of Depends you're wearing. Now, continue to sit in the wet brief for at least two hours. Not the way you want to end up, is it?)

Call them what you want …

The topic of Depends has historically been the subject of geriatric jokes or puns about infirmity. My good friend, in an effort to humor me, called them "party pants," a moniker she appropriated from stories of college girls rumored to wear them at wild drinking parties, concerts, and sporting events.

Out of the mouths of babes: After only one year of wearing Depends, my youngest daughter, who was eight at the time, told me that the term "party pants" didn't work anymore, since there was no party; and if there were, it definitely was over.

Thanks, sweetheart, for the reality check.

The sacral nerve stimulator

My neurologist directed me to the city's only urogynecologist—a physician who specialized in any combination of urological and gynecological issues for women—to whom she referred all her female MS patients with bladder problems.

After a lengthy consult, the urogynecologist decided I was a good candidate for an Inter-Stim, a surgically implanted sacral nerve stimulator. Applying select electrical impulses to the sacral nerve could reduce the frequency of my need to void and help empty my bladder more completely. I was immediately sold on the concept. I had the Inter-Stim surgically implanted in January 2005. It was placed in my lower right abdomen with its attached wires threaded through the sacral bone and placed up against the sacral nerves. The wires were programmed to mildly pulsate at designated frequencies to determine how often I urinated.

The Inter-Stim significantly reduced my need to pee from every three to four hours to every five to six hours and, therefore, cut the number of times I needed to complete my bathroom routine from six to four times each day. Although the device prolonged the time between bathroom breaks, over time its impact on the regularity of my voiding frequency diminished.

When I had difficulty with urine retention in 2008, the device failed to help empty my bladder; and, sadly, within three years, my MS worsened to the point that the device was unable to override the neurological damage to my bladder. My physician made several attempts to recalibrate the device's sensitivity, but its performance didn't improve as we desired. Disappointed, I deactivated the mechanism with my handheld remote control.

Why can't I have another MRI?

The three MRIs I had done in 1995, 1999, and 2002 were for current, updated looks at the MS lesions on my brain. Two of those MRIs were done with and without gadolinium contrast dye, which can indicate any new lesions that may have developed within the most recent six-week period. Both types of MRIs produced similar findings.

In 2006, my neurologist ordered an updated brain and spinal cord MRI, as well. While filling out the health intake form in the radiology department waiting room, I realized I needed to call Medtronic, the maker of the Inter-Stim, to check on the compatibility of an MRI with the Inter-Stim model I had implanted.

Fortunately, I checked this information, as Medtronic did *not* approve of patients with my Inter-Stim model having an MRI. This older version of the Inter-Stim, from early 2005, had the potential to cause internal burning with an MRI. Although an MRI was not firmly contraindicated with this model, the manufacturer strongly suggested that physicians inform their patients with these older sacral nerve stimulators not to have this radiographic exam because the safety risk was too high.

At the time of this writing, I am considering surgical removal of my Inter-Stim, a procedure my urogynecologist is said to have performed on numerous occasions. The removal of this older model will then allow me the benefit of having another MRI, this time, one of my spinal cord as well as my brain.

Something was wrong. Don't you hate it when you're right?

Blood spots randomly but persistently appeared on my Depends between November 2007 and April 2008. My PCAs and I believed, since I was perimenopausal, the source of blood was uterine.

When my father entered the critical end stage of bladder cancer with metastases and his health condition became a distraction from my own, I disregarded my "spotting issue" and didn't give it a second thought until he died in March 2008.

After his death, I was put on the toilet and an aide randomly collected a small trickle of my urine in a Dixie cup. Lo and behold, my bladder was the source of blood. I immediately called my primary care physician to report what we had found.

A nurse visited my home later that afternoon to collect a urine sample to send to the lab. My caregiver and I were shocked to see the large quantity of dark, "purple, grape-juice-colored urine," as the nurse described the catheterization sample in her nursing notes.

I had a mild fever that same evening, and although my temperature was only 98.6° F, this number was significantly higher than my normal temperature of 97.4° F. The next morning, my temperature was slightly higher at 99.4° F and was accompanied by low-grade, painful muscle stiffness; I was barely able to turn my neck. We anticipated that the results of my urine test would reveal bacteria, in addition to the blood, and the physician would declare a urinary tract infection.

The laboratory report results were shocking: no mention of the presence of either bacteria or blood in my urine. My family doctor deduced no urinary tract infection. Astoundingly, even my doctor's office had no comment about the nurse's documentation of the profound quantity of blood.

Because my physician thought there was no UTI, she didn't prescribe an antibiotic. Regardless of the lack of bacteria identified in the report, I remained convinced a UTI was in fact present. I presented my case for beginning empirical antibiotic treatment, and the doctor ordered Levaquin (levofloxacin), a powerful once-daily antibiotic.

I decided to visit a local hospital emergency room that evening for a computerized tomography (CT scan) of my bladder and another evaluation of my urine. I also wanted to check for the presence of kidney stones, which could be another aggravating cause of blood in my urine.

After he received my CT scan and a couple of blood and urine tests, the ER physician came to my examination room to review the results: "No lesions on your bladder, but your urine is full of bacteria," he announced.

Awkward. I think we've all been there. Your car engine is making clanking noises and screams for repair, but the moment you take it in to be fixed, it purrs like a kitten for the auto technician. The ER was ready to send me home, but I wasn't ready to go. Fortunately, my power of attorney called them and argued that I should be transferred to the hospital for further evaluation. I was admitted into the hospital, but my urine never did show signs of blood during that time. Perhaps I dreamt it.

Before I left the hospital, the attending urologist wrote me a prescription for Urecholine (bethanechol) for urinary retention. Although this older drug was effective at eliminating urine from my bladder, I experienced the frightening side effect of bronchospasm and found myself struggling to breathe while I was waiting in a grocery store aisle. There is no certain remedy for this except to discontinue use of the medication and wait until it has metabolized out of your system. I still sought emergency treatment; I was monitored closely and given a nebulizer with albuterol and Atrovent (ipratropium).

Here's where the story gets interesting!
Seven weeks after my hospital discharge, a personal-care aide and I were organizing my office and filing some loose documents. The mess of forgotten papers included the discharge summary from my most recent hospital visit.

I was interested in seeing the diagnoses indicated on my record, but instead I saw the words "Renal Ultrasound." I was stunned and fascinated. I had the same radiographic pictures taken of my bladder as they do of a pregnant woman's uterus. I had asked for the results but was never told what they were when I was released from the hospital.

I could hardly believe my eyes as I read the report test results and asked my PCA to repeat out loud what she saw written: "Renal Ultrasound: 2.5 cm mass located on posterior wall of bladder. ALERT: PATIENT TO FOLLOW UP WITH UROLOGY REGARDING ABNORMAL RENAL ULTRASOUND."

My PCA and I stood frozen with our mouths open and stared at each other in utter amazement. This dangerous oversight was shocking as not a single healthcare professional from all of those assigned to me at the hospital had mentioned this extremely important fact—not a nurse, not the urologist, not the ubiquitous hospitalist charged with overseeing the activity of my assigned physicians.

I contacted my urogynecologist immediately to follow up with the alarming notice of the growth in my bladder. Within a few days, I was sitting on her medieval-looking chair with an open bottom for conducting a cystoscopy.

The physician threaded the long skinny cable with a tiny camera mounted on one end through my urethra. She scanned the interior of my bladder with the photographic lens in search of the tumor. We saw it simultaneously. The growth appeared on the monitor and looked like a stalk of broccoli blossoming off the interior bladder wall. She biopsied the tumor tissue by clipping off a small sample and readied it to send to histology for examination.

Only a few days later, the doctor called me at home to inform me of the laboratory results: *positive for cancer.* I wasn't surprised by the news. Bladder cancer was most likely a consequence of my infrequent but persistent tobacco use for nearly thirty years. Also, my father, a former heavy smoker, had died of bladder cancer only three months earlier.

Removing the bladder tumor: The urologic oncologist

A urologic oncologist at The Ohio State University scheduled my surgery within two weeks and removed the tumor in July 2008. The interior surface of my bladder was immediately washed with mitomycin C, a chemotherapeutic drug in a topical solution. Fortunately, he characterized the removed tissue as "transitional cell" and "superficial and noninvasive." This is apparently a "good" cancer, although the term sounds oxymoronic.

Bladder won't empty: Nighttime catheterization, anyone?

During my first quarterly postsurgery cystoscopy follow-up, my urologic oncologist was alarmed that I was retaining 500–600 mL of urine in my bladder, calling it "an insane amount."

I told my urologist I felt that I fully emptied my bladder each time I peed. He disagreed, saying that the urine that left my bladder when I voided was merely "overflow," and I was not emptying the entire amount. He worried that too much remaining urine could back up through the ureters and place me at greater risk for kidney problems.[2]

He wanted me to have a Foley catheter inserted every evening and removed in the morning. His intention was to reduce the amount of urine I carried in my bladder at any one time during the day.

A nurse or a home-care attendant (HCA) visited my home each evening to catheterize me.[3] Awaiting her routine arrival each night made my schedule very inflexible, but the bothersome process proved to be a worthwhile effort. Wearing a catheter during the nighttime hours kept my buttocks dry from urine while I slept and produced a positive change to my butt's skin condition. Catheterization reduced

---

2 A 1964 review of autopsies of MS patients attributed 55 percent of deaths to hydronephrosis, swelling of the kidney due to backup of urine, or pyelonephritis, a kidney infection commonly caused by bacteria from the bladder. W. Samellas and B. Rubin, "Management of Upper Urinary Tract Complications in Multiple Sclerosis by Means of Urinary Diversion to an Ileal Conduit," *Journal of Urology* 93 (1965): 548.

3 In August 2010, the state of Ohio introduced the Home Care Attendant designation, which authorized personal-care aides to be trained and approved to conduct specific nursing tasks, including urinary catheterization.

the amount of residual urine during the day as if it had been retrained to hold less. After several months, the average amount of residual bladder urine had decreased to approximately 200 mL.

Routine urological equipment and catheter care

Although I was catheterized thirty times per month, I received only three Foley catheters, three urine drain bags, and three catheterization prep kits. The health insurance company would not pay for thirty of these supplies per month.

My urologist was unconcerned that sterile technique was not employed. He did not consider sterility (using boiled equipment) necessary and allowed sanitary or "clean technique" using soap and warm water.

Preventing urinary tract infections

The terms *bladder infection, cystitis,* and *UTI* are often used inter-changeably to describe an overpopulation of bacteria in this otherwise sterile environment. Bladder infections are most commonly identi-fied by symptoms of burning when urinating and lower abdominal cramping. Since MS has dulled these sensations for me, the first sign often includes fever and neck and arm stiffness with pain.

The most common cause of bladder infections is *Escherichia coli,* or E. coli, a type of bacteria that thrives in the lower colon and stool. If you're a woman, you have probably been repeatedly instructed to "wipe front to back" when cleaning the perineal area. This keeps the bacteria found near the rectum from populating the urethra and causing an infection.

Urinary catheters should be inserted and left in place no longer than absolutely essential and should not be used solely for the conve-nience of patient-care personnel.[4]

---

4 Centers for Disease Control, "National Nosocomial Infections Study Report," *Category I (Strongly Recommended for Adoption),* November 1979: 2–14.

Reported rates of urinary tract infections vary widely: a 1 to 5 percent incident rate after receiving a single brief catheterization,[5] but virtually 100 percent for patients wearing indwelling urethral catheters for longer than four days.[6]

Other ways to protect the urinary tract from infection

As a prophylactic measure to prevent UTIs, my urologist prescribes the antibiotic Macrobid (nitrofurantoin) 50 mg once each day. Macrobid is a relatively safe medication whose course runs primarily through the urine. Since I have been taking this medicine, I have not had a single episode of bacterial infection in my urinary tract.

Drinking cranberry juice has long been thought to be a great deterrent against UTIs, but a recent meta-analysis of at least ten different well-designed research studies concluded differently.[7]

Urinary tract infection: How do I know if I have one?

When I didn't have MS and could easily identify abdominal cramping, I could sense when I had a UTI. If I had a burning sensation when I peed, frequent urination, cloudy urine, and a dull, continuous achy lower abdominal area, I knew I was in trouble.

Now the most suspicious warning signs of a UTI include an increase in muscle stiffness and body temperature. When I experience both of these symptoms, I usually call my physician to have my urine tested.

Quick overview of bladder control

Treat your bladder with respect: it can be a source of harmony or hell.

---

5 M. Turck, B. Goffe, and R. G. Petersdorf, "The Urethral Catheters and Urinary Tract Infection," *Journal of Urology* 88 (1962): 834–37.

6 E. H. Kass, "Asymptomatic Infections of the Urinary Tract," *Transactions of the Association of American Physicians* 69 (1956):56–63.

7, C.-H. Wang, et al., "Cranberry-Containing Products for Prevention of Urinary Tract Infections in Susceptible Populations: A Systematic Review and Meta-analysis of Randomized Controlled Trials," *Archives of Internal Medicine* 172, no. 13 (2012): 988–96; doi:10.1001/archinternmed.2012.3004.

Regardless of whether or not a catheter is needed, be careful not to introduce bacteria around or inside the orifice of the urethra. Recognize that the most common bacteria that causes bladder infections is E. coli from the lower colon.

If catheterization is needed, minimize the duration of use to only what is necessary for eliminating the contents of the bladder. Intermittent catheterization, although done multiple times each day, is less likely to cause a UTI than an indwelling catheter, which is inserted into the urethra only once. Although preliminary data on the risk of infection are encouraging, the benefit of the suprapubic catheter with regard to incidence of infections has not been clearly proven.

I drink fluids as consistently as possible during the day. A beverage holder is mounted to an armrest on my wheelchair with a long straw. Although pure water would be the best choice, I favor a mixed beverage of half cranberry juice and half sparkling water.

My urine drain bag is checked every morning to monitor the color and clarity of my urine. If I have consumed adequate fluids, the color of my urine should be light yellow with no sediment. If urine is amber in color, this could mean I consumed too little fluid and need to increase the amount.

Dealing with the bladder is a necessary evil

Adults negotiate who will change the baby's next diaper. Potty training is a rite of passage, and despite the freedom of a child's newfound independence, the little person still requires assistance in the bathroom.

People have different thresholds for "holding it" and what they consider private enough circumstances for urinating in public, as evidenced by the spectrum of answers to the question during car trips: "Can you wait until the next exit, or would you rather just pee on the side of the road?"

No matter our age or health condition, where to pee will always remain a predicament in our lives.

Chapter 7
Battle Between Brain and Brawn: Spasticity

Muscle weakness and loss of balance were my first symptoms of MS, but soon after, unusually tense muscles in my arms and legs began to set in. My stiff, uncooperative body became more than just an annoyance, and it took concentrated effort to stay erect as I walked. Even while sitting down and relaxing, just lifting one leg and crossing it over the other was complicated. Reaching to grab a can of pop was a challenge. Muscle spasticity made all my appendages—legs, arms, hands, and fingers—stiff and noncompliant.

Uncontrollable muscle tightening was aggravating. Whenever I needed to move, my arms and legs would inconveniently "lock up" and reject any attempt I made to straighten or bend them. Walking up a set of stairs required hooking a feeble arm around my thigh and trying to lift it high enough for my foot to reach the next step. I was no longer in command of how my body moved; it was in control of me.

Spasticity results from a battle between flexor and extensor muscles. Flexor muscles want to contract and shorten to form a fist, while extensor muscles stretch and elongate.

Spasticity held me back from moving around at the speed to which I was accustomed prior to MS. As time progressed, even holding a hairbrush and reaching the back of my head was becoming impossible to do. My muscles would tighten no matter how hard I tried to get them to loosen up. It was frustrating to know my functional abilities were declining. Emotional stress from not being able to take action only made things worse. My saying was, "The faster I try to go, the slower I become." Remaining seated in a rigid position was easier than any effort to transfer out of it.

Slinging my legs up onto the surface of the bed at night was an arduous process. Even with the use of a long, rigid, hand-controlled "leg lift" with a foot strap at the bottom, I still had to apply quite a bit of determined physical and mental effort into catapulting them from one position to another.

The muscle tightness in my legs increased so much that I could hardly spread them apart with two hands. At a gynecology exam I joked about needing to loosen the vice grip of my thighs with a crowbar. I found separating them was essential for cleaning my "whosywhatsit."

Problems with muscle spasticity began in my legs but gradually traveled to my upper extremities. I began to notice that combined muscle tightness and weakening migrated to my hands and fingers when I could barely hold the scissors and my son's hair for a cut. I didn't have enough strength to raise my arms or spread my fingers wide enough apart to grab a thin section of his hair or to hold the hair straight between my index and middle fingers. I couldn't hold a pen securely or write legibly in smooth, steady movements. Grasping the knob on the handicapped driver's wheel of my van became a rough and eventually impossible endeavor.

The benefit of physical therapy

My neurologist ordered an evaluation by a physical therapist (PT). This would be the first of five PTs assigned to me over the next fourteen years. Each one was charged with developing an exercise regimen that suited my changing physical needs.

Every three to four years my physical therapy requirements evolved, and each time I was assigned to a new therapist. The first therapist concentrated on strengthening the core muscles of my trunk and instructed me to sit on a large, inflatable rubber ball to increase strength needed to balance my body. The second PT focused on maintaining my ability to stand straight by walking me through a set of parallel bars without relying on them for support. The third PT conducted her professional calls at my home and developed an exercise plan that integrated use of my bedroom furniture—squats and leg lifts holding on to the footboard of my bed and carrying out other miscellaneous calisthenics while lying on my bed. The fourth therapist developed a workout program that deferred any strength training to my arms only and limited stretching and range-of-motion exercises to my legs.

I finally lost the ability to use both my legs and arms and was enrolled as a "consumer" in the Ohio Home Care Program. In addition to being provided personal-care assistance for most of each day, a physical therapist also started visiting my home once a week ad infinitum, unlike prior PT coverage with my private insurer, which was limited to a twelve-week maximum service period.

I have been with my present physical therapists for four years. He reduced my scope of therapy to passive exercise and stretching only. He focuses on the importance of my remaining limber and without contractures (permanent shortening of muscles).

To optimize my flexibility, each personal-care aide is instructed to engage me in range-of-motion exercises. A variety of motions to help keep every joint in my body "lubricated"—starting with my shoulders, arms, wrists, and fingers and progressing to my hip joints, knees, ankles, and toes—is posted on a bulletin board for all to see.

When exercising with any of my five physical therapists, I was never overexerted and always encouraged to taper back from any physical demands at the point of fatigue. Active exercise is beneficial but can be counterproductive if exhaustion drains me mentally and prevents me from further movement.

Involuntary spasticity triggers

Some involuntary movements can exacerbate spasticity. Other stimuli, such as yawning and transferring, can also be triggers for a tightening of the muscles.[1] Whenever I am repositioned in my bed first

1 A. Shah and I. Maitlin, "Spasticity Due to Multiple Sclerosis: Epidemiology, Pathophysiology, and Treatment," chap. 22, in *Spasticity: Diagnosis and Management,* ed. by A. Brashear and E. Elovic (New York: Demos Medical Publishing, 2010).

thing in the morning or yawn wildly, no one dares to attempt to move my body any further because I freeze up, and all my muscles become obstinate. Whenever I would hold my youngest daughter's hand, she would plead with me not to yawn so the muscles in my hands would not squeeze hers tightly in the process!

Use of baclofen tablets for spasticity
Baclofen (lioresal) is the cornerstone medication for antispasticity therapy. I have used this medication for relief from muscle cramping and tightness for more than thirteen years. Baclofen counteracts the stimulating action (producing an inhibitory effect) on flexor muscles resulting in a gentle muscle relaxation. [Baclofen is unrelated to other more powerful muscle relaxers like Flexeril (cyclobenzaprine) or Soma (carisoprodol), which involve additional compounds produced by the body and are associated with sedation.]

Baclofen tablets were given at least three times each day. During the night, when the intensity of my muscle spasms became greatest, I had to be awakened to receive an overnight dose for relief. This useful drug can cause dizziness and drowsiness, but I never experienced these side effects.

To keep my muscles relaxed and without spasticity, I found myself needing at least one baclofen 10 mg oral tablet every four to six hours during the day and once in the middle of the night. I took a total of 40 mg every day within the first few months of my diagnosis and stayed on the same dose for about seven years.

As my spasticity grew worse over the next few years, I found myself seeking relief from closer to 80 mg a day. My physiatrist, a rehabilitation physician, increased my dose to 100 mg but said I could increase it to 120 mg if absolutely necessary. However, it seemed that I had reached an effectiveness plateau. Doses higher than 40 mg daily didn't offer any additional relief. Once, I tried samples of another medication for spasticity, Zanaflex (tizanidine), but did not find it to be as effective for muscle spasms as baclofen.

Gabapentin for spasticity

Gabapentin first came on the pharmaceutical market as Neurontin. The FDA originally approved this medication for treatment of seizures. It was so weak at controlling seizure activity, however, that it could be prescribed only in combination with another antiseizure medication and wasn't often recommended for this condition. Soon, gabapentin was being prescribed for off-label uses, including spasticity.

When I visited a neurologist at the Cleveland Clinic in 2003 for another opinion of my MS treatment, I complained of a slight burning, itchy feeling on the bottoms of my feet. She interpreted this as an indicator of peripheral neuropathy and prescribed gabapentin at bedtime for its stabilizing effect on nerve membranes.

I didn't fill the gabapentin prescription for two reasons: one, the itchy, burning sensation in my feet disappeared (these symptoms only bothered me for one day), and two, I felt that I was accumulating far too many medications for someone my age.

Six months later, I serendipitously discovered medical literature citing gabapentin for use in spasticity. The references inspired me to see whether the medication could help relieve my spasticity not controlled by baclofen alone.

Surprisingly, gabapentin helped me limber up and allowed me to draw my knees toward my abdomen and roll out of bed in the morning. Although gabapentin can cause drowsiness, it didn't cause any additional sleepiness for me. I experimented with baclofen alone versus baclofen and gabapentin and found that the combination was more effective than either drug by itself for spasticity.

Botox therapy

Botox is well known as a popular cosmetic treatment for facial wrinkling, but what most people don't realize is that Botox (botulism toxin) was developed and first used as a therapeutic treatment for muscle spasms. Somebody at a clinical laboratory somewhere woke up one day with an awesome idea to find another way to maximize the use of this agent for a profitable and valuable purpose. Injections of very small amounts of the toxin produced by the same bacteria that cause botulism are used to relax tight muscles on the face. It wasn't until Botox was used for this cosmetic application that it gained such worldwide recognition. (I hope the person who moved the world forward with this clever idea is enjoying a happy, early retirement today.)

Despite daily range-of-motion exercises, the muscles in my hands and fingers were always contracted. Baclofen and gabapentin oral therapy were producing marginal relaxation in these muscles, but I wanted a more aggressive antispasticity regimen. My physiatrist suggested Botox therapy.

This therapy consisted of intramuscular injections placed into the area of the extensor muscle that refused to relax. One session of Botox therapy consisted of eighteen uncomfortable injections inserted at different sites throughout the muscles in my arms, hands, and thumbs.

Botox therapy greatly reduced the amount of tension in my arm and hand muscles. My personal care aides immediately noticed a difference in their ability to move my appendages more easily when bathing, transferring, and dressing me.

Personally, I had hoped to relax the muscles in my hands enough to cause them to lie flat on my arm rests and was disappointed that this did not occur. I realized that my desire to use Botox therapy was merely for aesthetic reasons. I needed to reevaluate the "pain-to-gain ratio" of using Botox for this purpose. Although I was having difficulty rationalizing another round of botulism toxin injections, I decided to give this therapy another try.

Four months later, I succumbed to the next sequence of Botox injections. But this time, my physiatrist actually increased the number of shots to twenty-two with the hope of enhancing the medication's therapeutic effect.

The second round of Botox therapy did not provide a worthwhile outcome either. Once again, my aides were impressed at how well this medication produced muscle compliance, but I wasn't as impressed because my expectations for this "cosmetic" medication to give me a "cosmetic" advantage were not met. I decided the results of Botox therapy were not worth the pain and discontinued further use.

Electric stimulation therapy (eStim)

My next appointment with the physiatrist was in the electromyography lab at The Ohio State University's physical medicine department. I shared my unfavorable assessment of my Botox experience with him.

He knew I was radically closed-minded about having an intrathecal baclofen pump surgically implanted as he had recommended. So, instead of readdressing what could be a moot discussion, he changed his strategy and demonstrated electrical stimulation (eStim) therapy. He firmly pressed a probe to the skin on my upper forearm (at the insertion point for the muscles in my hand) to activate the nerve below that controlled my fingers.

Seeing a single finger receive a jolt and pop up out of alignment with the other fingers was like watching a magician pull a rabbit out of a hat! I was amazed and terribly encouraged by the application of eStim to control my muscles. My physiatrist ordered this therapy with a physical therapist three times each week for six weeks.

I called to schedule the series of appointments with the physical therapy (PT) department but was rerouted to the occupational therapy (OT) department, instead. I was told by the appointment desk that OT typically takes care of rehabilitation issues from "the elbow down to the hands and fingers," and PT deals with issues involving the "elbows up and the rest of the body."

The notion that the application of eStim could put a muscle into motion was fantastic. I was excited to start the therapy, but unfortunately, the eStim unit used by the OT department produced a considerably weaker effect than the one the physiatrist had demonstrated.

The OT department used an eStim machine that had only several dime-sized, flat electronic patches instead of a long electrical probe. The physiatrist used the single metal probe with great accuracy in identifying a specific point of the muscle to be stimulated. But, when the occupational therapist tried to control the movement of one finger, the lower strength eStim machine seemed to merely irritate a cluster of nonspecific nerves located under a small spot on my skin, making my entire hand budge sluggishly.

Originally, I had high hopes for eStim therapy. After the lackluster results I received from this portable device, however, I had to reconsider whether continuing this therapy made sense. Although the medical facility was only twenty minutes from my home, I needed to evaluate the amount of time, energy, and car expense required to prepare for and travel to three appointments each week.

I decided to go for one more round of eStim therapy, but it was likely going to end anyway. My occupational therapist informed me that, to continue eStim therapy, the health insurance company required documentation of a functional improvement from the therapy.

My hands didn't seem to benefit much from this therapy. Out of desperation the therapist wrapped my fingers around a spoon so I could pick up plastic "cereal" pieces from a bowl and lift them up and into my mouth as evidence that the eStim therapy improved my ability to feed myself. This effort was futile, and therapy was discontinued.

The limitations of the electrical stimulation device proved to be the last time I would attempt to improve my muscular functioning. From that day on, I lost all confidence in the ability of any intervention—physical or chemical—to help retrain or possibly reactivate muscles. I stopped searching for remedies to do so.

Scoliosis caused by spasticity?

I visited an orthopedic physician's office in 2005 for a strained rotator cuff and received treatment with an intra-articular injection of cortisone. It was brought to my doctor's attention that one shoulder drooped significantly lower than the other as I sat in my wheelchair. He lifted up the back of my shirt and followed the length of my spine from the back of my head to my tailbone with his finger pressed firmly over the skin covering my bony spinal structure.

About halfway down the length of my back was an obvious C

curve in the spine. The doctor determined that I had scoliosis. I had never been diagnosed with this back anomaly, even as a young girl in elementary school, so it's doubtful it was congenital. I was eager to explore causes for scoliosis to appear later in my life.

At that point the only significant change in my health had been MS, and I was interested in knowing whether it played any role. Although neuromuscular diseases, in general, are mentioned as probable causes of scoliosis, I found no firm research about the relationship between MS and this condition. There were references indicating that scoliosis-like curvatures occurred with cerebral palsy. The intervertebral muscles on one side of my spine might have become spastic and pulled the spinal column tightly to the same side, making this shoulder appear lower than the other and causing a visual curve to appear on the other side.

The orthopedic physician did not accept my theory about spastic muscles with MS causing this spinal curvature. Within the year, however, my shoulder height became more symmetrical and signs of scoliosis barely detectable. Could it be that the muscle spasms relaxed?

The intrathecal baclofen pump: Tell me more

When OT therapy with the electrical stimulation unit ended, I reconsidered receiving another round of Botox injections. I revisited the notion of whether or not the benefit of getting numerous injections had outweighed the pain.

The occupational therapist convinced me before I left her service to seriously consider a baclofen pump. She had worked with a number of patients with spastic muscles who had been successfully managed with an intrathecal baclofen pump and thought I might be a good candidate for one as well.

In theory, a baclofen pump made perfect sense and seemed a viable alternative to more Botox. A constant amount of baclofen, the medication used to relieve the tight, uncomfortable muscular spasticity, could be delivered in a constant dose directly into the spinal cord fluid sac, using a fraction of the baclofen I consumed orally. But

I wanted to avoid surgical implantation of a drug pump for as long as possible.

My concerns were quirky and perhaps invalid; but because I worked as a pharmacist in the 1980s, I had an old-fashioned, closet fear of these mechanical devices. When they first came on the market, I recall the detailed calculations required to determine the total pump refill amount and to program the rate of drug delivery accurately. Early on, there was a mystique associated with these robotic instruments whose purpose was to supply the body with a steady amount of morphine and fentanyl to treat intractable, malignant pain. Talk of "runaway pumps," dose dumping, and locating a qualified healthcare professional to refill them led to heady discussions.

It made me queasy to think I needed a grueling surgery to implant a second Medtronic pump, this time in the opposite side of my abdominal cavity, and lay a catheter within the delicate interior space surrounding my spinal cord. However, I decided to rid myself of any preconceived notions from thirty years ago that might be holding me back from making an educated decision about intrathecal pumps. I brought myself up to date by watching a DVD my physiatrist encouraged me to view.

During an office appointment, the surgeon who would implant a baclofen pump had invited a satisfied MS patient into the examination room. The young man in his thirties could not stop talking about how much the drug pump had improved his quality of life. Truthfully, the conversation with him made me think more favorably about the whole idea.

The notion of a surgically placed intrathecal pump still scared me. I tried to gather thoughts of a catheter in more positive light to help quell my fears about the surgery. To distract me from my fear of risky spinal surgery, I concentrated on the advantage: not needing a dose of oral baclofen every four to six hours and in the middle of the night.

Actually, my dark sense of humor finally prompted my decision. I asked myself a rhetorical question: Why am I worried about the potential danger of paraplegia? Why do I care if this surgery prevents me from walking again? Hmm.

The Medtronic intrathecal pump is shaped like a large hockey puck and filled with a sterile solution of baclofen. This internal titanium pump was surgically implanted into my left lower abdomen with the catheter running upward through the spine and finally inserted into the T-3 vertebral area of the spinal cord.

Now I require only 139 mcg (0.139 mg) each day intrathecally versus 80 mg orally. This lower intrathecal amount calculates to less than 0.17 percent of the original oral baclofen dose I was taking by mouth. Because the intrathecal medication is not absorbed by the stomach, it bypasses the liver, and a much smaller dose of baclofen is utilized by the body. Less baclofen in the bloodstream translates to fewer side effects, including drowsiness. The baclofen pump provides continuous relief from muscle spasms, which can range from bothersome to painful.

The surgery was incident free. The nurse from Medtronic was on hand at the hospital the same day as my surgery to evaluate any starting dose adjustments. Several hours after surgery, it was already apparent that I required a baclofen dosing adjustment; the muscles in my back and arms were tight and uncomfortable. An order was given to the Medtronic nurse in the hospital to modify the pump's programming and slowly increase the amount of baclofen delivered to the intrathecal space.

I didn't observe an instant difference between the oral dose of baclofen and the intrathecal therapy. Over a few-week period, however, the new smoother dosing with the baclofen pump eliminated the drug level fluctuations that either made me too tired or too stiff when I took the oral tablets.

The baclofen pump requires refills with the commercially prepared drug solution about every four months. My physiatrist's nurse palpates my abdomen to identify the location of the tiny opening of the pump. Then she inserts a long needle filled with baclofen liquid; surprisingly, it doesn't hurt.

As reluctant as I was to have an intrathecal baclofen pump, I am terribly pleased that I agreed to receive one. The most remarkable improvement has been the steady drug level and my ability to sleep through the night without being awakened by muscle spasms and relying on an additional oral dose of baclofen for relief. The pump ultimately reduced my dependence on a caregiver to come to my home during the middle of the night to give me my medicine. The benefit of more complete spasticity control has certainly outweighed any negative concerns that were holding me back.

Chapter 8
MS Just Wasn't Enough, Apparently: Trigeminal Neuralgia

The probability of having trigeminal neuralgia (TN)—the nerve disorder that causes God-awful stabbing pain in the face—is low. The incidence of TN has been reported as only 4.3 people per 100,000 population.[1]

The odds of having MS are also low, reported to be between 1 in 1,200 to 1,500 people. Out of this very small group of individuals, however, up to 2 percent will also have TN.[2] I was among that tiny 2 percent. (Hitting those uncommon numbers with such low odds, I might do well at playing the lottery.)

TN is also referred to as tic douloureux.[3] "Suicide disease" is another term loosely mentioned in literature. This moniker grabbed my attention because I could easily understand how a person could wish herself dead in a desperate attempt to stop the grisly pain. Many times I refused to drink or eat to avoid triggering the excruciating, electric-shock-like jabs.

The pathophysiology of this painful facial syndrome is believed to be a result of a pulsating cerebellar artery rubbing against one of the three branches of the large fifth cranial nerve, the trigeminal nerve. In MS, however, TN is thought to be due to plaque formation that damages and irritates that same nerve.

An ironclad diagnosis of TN is difficult to make. The questionable

---

1   S. Katusic, C. M. Beard, E. Bergstralh, and L. T. Kurland, "Incidence and Clinical Features of Trigeminal Neuralgia," Rochester, Minnesota, 1945–1984, *Annals of Neurology* 27, no. 1 (1990): 89–95.

2   J. P. Hooge and W. K. Redekop, "Trigeminal Neuralgia with Multiple Sclerosis," *Neurology* 45 (1995): 1294–96.

3   R. P. Rapini, J. L. Bolognia, and J. L. Jorizzo, *Dermatology* (St. Louis: Mosby, 2007), 101.

source of pain can baffle dental and medical practitioners alike. And because the pain is so similar to that of an abscessed tooth, patients have been known to request extraction of perfectly healthy teeth.

The trigeminal nerve is both a sensory and motor nerve. Because cranial nerves originate in the brain rather than the spinal cord, they are often considered part of the central nervous system as opposed to the peripheral nervous system. The intense sensation of pain is unlike any I've ever known.

The intensity of the maddening jolts of pain from TN is nearly impossible to define. The trigeminal nerve, when irritated, produces a profound lightning-shock sensation, as if I had sucked on a live electric wire. Labor and contractions with three childbirths and three root canals were mild compared to the agony of TN.

How my trigeminal neuralgia was finally diagnosed

I sensed several worrisome pangs in my upper molars over a three- to four-year period without any clue as to what was going on. The feeling resembled what I had experienced from my first pre-root canal surgery thirty-five years before. At my next dental appointment, a dental student determined that I needed a filling for a large cavity that had decayed through the dentin, tunneled far into an upper back molar, and was perilously close to the nerve root below.

Despite receiving a new amalgam filling for this molar, I continued to have stabbing pain in the upper back portion, or maxillary area, of my mouth. The dentist supervisor at The Ohio State University dental school suspected my discomfort might be a sign of fibromyalgia associated with my MS. We also talked about the possibility of deafferentation, a type of pain resulting from interruption of nerve impulses.

A year later, the same area around the upper right molar throbbed periodically and progressively grew worse, I returned to the Advanced Endodontic Clinic, or "tooth pain clinic." An endodontic student conducted an evaluation of my tooth with a digital x-ray. Because she detected erosion through the cavity floor, she proceeded to perform a root canal on the tooth.

The day after the root canal, the familiar pain rebounded, and I went back once again to the same endodontic student to double-check that no residual decay lurked around the roots of the affected molar. Although there was no sign of tooth abscess on the x-ray, the endodontic student subtly questioned her own procedure and chose to repeat the root canal for good measure.

The day after her encore root canal on the same molar, the sharp, penetrating shocks emanating from the upper maxillary region persisted. Mortified about being unable to tolerate the pain, I returned to the dental school and was seen this time by a first-year male endodontic student.

After two root canals on the same tooth, the horrific pain refused to go away, but the digital x-ray failed to reveal any structural defect. I was terribly confused and embarrassed, and the student appeared bored and unconvinced while I rambled on about this maddening, mysterious pain in my mouth. I pleaded for options to help direct my next move. Despite conferring with his supervisor, he only offered two alternatives: do nothing or remove the tooth.

If those were my only two choices, I thought, the decision was an easy one: "Get rid of it."

Within an hour, I was being processed as a patient in the oral surgery department one floor above. Even after the area surrounding the tooth was completely anesthetized and the permanent molar was extracted, an odd foreboding twinge remained in the same upper palate area on the right side of my mouth.

Pulling out the huge tooth had a paradoxical effect: Instead of the expected relief, my mouth pain and misery intensified. The extraction created a cavernous hole where there should have been a tooth and the new hollow seemed to expose the ultrasensitive nerves. I contacted my primary care physician immediately, desperate for help. She ordered a CT scan of my mouth to rule out a possible maxillary sinus infection.

The med tech from my doctor's office called the next day with the results of my CT scan. The results were negative for a maxillary sinus infection; therefore, no antibiotic was needed. To break through her matter-of-fact attitude, I forcefully reminded her that I was still in a fantastic amount of pain. I am not proud to admit it, but I actually yelled at her, freely peppering my complaints with profanity. "What the hell am I supposed to do?" I screamed. "I'm in a lot of f***ing pain!!!"

The poor girl had only been working with my physician a couple of weeks and was already being screamed at by some hysterical woman for no apparent reason—at least not for anything she had done. I'm sure she was stunned. I felt terrible for taking out my anger on her, but no one was listening and nothing else was working. Diplomacy certainly wasn't. My physician ordered an antibiotic to hedge against a potential subclinical sinus infection.

I took the antibiotic for a couple of days, but it did nothing to lessen the pain. Desperate, I popped a couple of leftover Vicodin (hydrocodone) from an old root canal prescription I had stored in my medicine cabinet. The drug did nothing to lessen the intensity of my torment.

The only effective healing agent turned out to be time. As the weeks passed, and the post-extraction crater in my mouth shrank, the pain slowly subsided. I was relieved. Within six months, however, the sneaky pain had reemerged, and I needed to visit the tooth pain clinic for yet another evaluation of severe "tooth" pain. This time, the pain radiated from the same side of my mouth, but it was now concentrated on a lower back molar.

I received a digital dental x-ray from a new endodontic student and was told there was no sign of decay. The student feared drilling the tooth and finding "a perfectly healthy nerve." Reluctantly, I agreed. Suspecting an imminent return to the dental clinic, I demanded one of her business cards with her direct phone line so I could call her if the pain returned.

Surprisingly, four months passed before I made another trip to the tooth clinic. Again, the digital x-ray was negative for tooth abscess. By this time, I was beginning to suspect the pain was not from my teeth and asked the endodontic student whether my pain could possibly be from trigeminal neuralgia or a temporomandibular joint disorder (TMJ).

My jaw made a loud "popping" noise when I chewed even small bites of food, a classic sign of TMJ. But as distracting as this was, it had never caused me pain. I recalled becoming aware of trigeminal neuralgia when I was a consultant pharmacist evaluating pharmaceutical care in a long-term care environment. I began to wonder if my clinical state was consistent with the criteria of this diagnosis.

The endodontic student who was advising me said it was possible to have either of these conditions and referred me to my neurologist. This turned out to be a godsend. In my experience, a clinician may feel reluctant to send a patient to another healthcare provider for a second opinion, so I was genuinely relieved to hear this dentist admit that she could not find a link between my facial pain and my teeth.

Seeing my neurologist for possible TN

I rambled on, describing my dental/medical case to the neurologist *in chronological detail* to help her make a diagnosis. It didn't take much beyond what I had said to convince her that I was suffering from trigeminal neuralgia.

Management of trigeminal neuralgia often begins with anticonvulsant medications, which act as nerve membrane stabilizers to control the transmission of pain. The drug of choice for TN is Tegretol (carbamazepine) out of a host of other drugs including baclofen and gabapentin, which are generally used to control seizures and spasticity.

I was already using gabapentin 300 mg twice daily and had a baclofen intrathecal pump running at 139 mcg per day for spasticity. Because I had outrageous pain despite doses of these medications, my neurologist opted to increase my gabapentin to 600 mg three times each day. Unfortunately, even the higher doses of gabapentin did absolutely nothing to lessen my discomfort.

The first round of carbamazepine proved to be effective in providing pain relief from TN, but it came at a cost. Carbamazepine made me lethargic. I slept an extra four to five hours each day, my speech was slurred, and I found it difficult to enunciate clearly and audibly. I deliberately concentrated on how I spoke and made certain my words were correctly interpreted by my computer's voice-recognition software.

In short, carbamazepine rated poorly on my quality-of-life scale, but, since no other drug came close to controlling the pain, it became a necessary evil. I tried using higher doses of carbamazepine but didn't experience any additional pain relief. I was becoming suspicious that the generic manufacturer had failed to put the active ingredient in the tablet, but the reality was that I was experiencing tolerance to the drug.

Anything I put in my mouth with flavor would set off a reaction in my salivary glands and initiate a pain response so that eventually I preferred not to eat at all. I diluted oatmeal with plenty of milk to keep it bland and to blend it into a fine consistency suitable for sucking through a straw, which I placed on the side of my mouth where I didn't have TN pain.

A nerve block of the trigeminal V3 nerve

My neurologist wasn't ready to discuss surgical intervention until all "medical management" attempts to control the pain had been exhausted. I wasn't interested in suffering for an undetermined length of time trying drugs with questionable effectiveness for TN. Plus, anticonvulsant therapy with nerve membrane stabilizers had notorious side effects, and I wanted to avoid them.

I contacted the physician who had surgically placed my intrathecal baclofen pump because I knew he was also a pain-management specialist. He offered to perform a nerve block on the affected branch of the trigeminal nerve responsible for my pain.

I was scheduled for the nerve block within a week and was anxious to feel relief from the agony that wouldn't let me concentrate on anything else. At the hospital I was prepped for surgery and rolled on a hospital bed into a well-lit operating room. My body was unable to remain still during the painful procedure because I was not under general anesthesia nor completely sedated. Instead, I was given a small amount of IV Versed (midazolam)—a benzodiazepine similar to Valium (diazapam)—to relax me throughout the procedure. The doctor's reason for keeping me awake was to make sure I was conscious enough to identify the targeted TN branch. To accomplish this, he relied on my somatic reactions to being jabbed on the right side of my face with a needle.

The doctor tried to locate each branch of my trigeminal nerve and single out V3, where the pain seemed to originate. Once identified, he would inject that nerve with the anesthetic Marcaine (bupivicaine). The series of wicked stabs to the skin of my face I endured while the doctor tried to locate the correct branch of my trigeminal nerve was distressing.

Because no radiographic equipment was used to navigate through the convoluted network of neurons in this procedure, the doctor judged the location of my body's anatomic structures by how I responded when touched in various locations. He associated the location of each TN branch by the response to the pricks of the individual facial muscles. For example, the V1 nerve that surrounds the ocular section would cause my eyebrow muscle to spasm; and V2, which covers the maxillary area, would cause my upper lip to quiver. There was no doubt where V3 was located. I wanted to shoot to the moon to escape the tormenting pain whenever pressure was applied to it.

The pain of the nerve block procedure was indescribable, and I had hoped my martyr-like effort to cooperate wasn't in vain. My physician warned me that I might not get the results I desired because I flinched my head often while he tried to administer the anesthetizing drug.

Whether we missed the V3 mark with Marcaine or the drug therapy was ineffective, the pain-free bliss, unfortunately, lasted less than three weeks. The TN pain returned, and I worked furiously to find a physician who could conduct a different type of surgery for TN.

My (first) rhizotomy on V3

I could not find any physician who claimed to specialize in trigeminal neuralgia, but finally I was referred to a young French Canadian neurosurgeon at The Ohio State University who specialized in neurovascular surgery. At our first meeting, he explained that surgical treatments for TN involved interfering with the most likely cause of the nerve pain. When a nerve and artery might be rubbing against each other, one method is to insert a small piece of Teflon between the aggravated trigeminal nerve and the offending artery. For patients with MS, however, plaque formation on the trigeminal nerve was deemed more likely to be the irritating factor. Therefore, the use of percutaneous radiofrequency rhizotomy to burn and "deaden" the irritated nerve tissue was expected to produce the best results.

Since I was contraindicated for an MRI, the neurosurgeon guesstimated my trigeminal neuralgia was most likely caused by damage from MS plaque formation. Using rhizotomy to destroy the nerve seemed to be the best treatment.

I was placed on my neurosurgeon's busy schedule for a surgery date and had no choice but to wait two grueling weeks. I restarted carbamazepine therapy in the meantime to help keep the pain at bay. Unfortunately, I had developed tolerance to the medication, and this round was much less effective than the first. I received a higher dose of carbamazepine for relief, but it was like my body was saying, "Sorry, not this time."

The pain of trigeminal neuralgia took my breath away and could not be controlled with even narcotic analgesics such as Vicodin (hydrocodone) and Percocet (oxycodone). Funny how pain can force people to do things they normally wouldn't do. I termed carbamazepine the "stupid drug" because of its lethargic and sedating side effects and swore I would never take another dose of it … at least not until the pain reoccurred. But once I realized how badly I needed relief, I was quick to forget my commitment and restarted therapy with this medication. (I freely confess that I would make a pathetic "sellout" prisoner of war and couldn't be trusted. I would probably reveal valuable secrets to the enemy in exchange for freedom from torture.)

My day in the hospital finally arrived, and my prayers were answered by a rhizotomy to interrupt communication between the damaged facial trigeminal nerve and the brain. I was comfortably medicated, but not asleep, during the procedure that was destroying the aggravating nerve. The entire process lasted only minutes and involved a quick piercing through the skin on my right cheek with a searing hot metal probe that used high-frequency radio waves.

Once the surgery was completed, I was rolled out of the operating room and into the recovery room. Strangely, I didn't feel complete relief. Soon after the mild anesthesia wore off, I could sense the silent threat of pain looming. Within three days, my facial nerves became even more unstable and explosive than they had been before the rhizotomy. What went wrong? Not only had the pain not abated, but my trigeminal neuralgia was escalating to new heights. Wasn't this madness supposed to end?

The (second) rhizotomy on V2 and V3

The neurosurgeon and I agreed that the new, uncontrollable pain was most likely from the V2 trigeminal nerve we hadn't considered to be the problem. This unfathomable pain occurred without warning as if V2 was retaliating for the senseless killing of a close family member, V3. A second rhizotomy, this time for both V2 and V3 nerves, was scheduled.

I was readmitted to the hospital and vigilantly avoided even the slightest muscle movement or brushing of the skin on my face, as they could easily bring on ballistic pain. I remained in a fetal position, knowing it was safer to sleep away the hours than to be awake. I prayed to God to drive away the evil pain spirits as I counted the minutes until the Tuesday after a long, harrowing Labor Day weekend.

My clenched jaw muscles and grinding teeth could initiate the excruciating pain, and I was haunted by IV morphine's inability to control it. Because I knew this powerful narcotic didn't work for me, I wanted to try Ativan (lorazepam) to preserve my sanity until my next rhizotomy surgery.

Some healthcare practitioners have a stellar academic standing but "sucky" bedside manner and people skills. Sadly, I was the victim of an insensitive night-shift medical resident who applied a textbook procedure and disregarded quality of life. I couldn't open my mouth for an oral dose of medication and, given my severe apprehension, wanted an injectable dose of Ativan (lorazepam) to muffle my interior screaming and intense muscle clenching. I wasn't even able to whisper, and I could barely form the words "Ativan IV" with my lips. When the physician finally understood what I was asking for, he immediately scolded me, "Ativan *is not* for pain, Ms. Wolf. Now, open your mouth so you can take these carbamazepine tablets." (Silly me for thinking I still had clinical collaboration power—especially as a mute. I'm sure the arrogant, young doctor was convinced he had taught me a valuable pharmacology lesson.)

I remained defiant and kept my eyes shut, tears squeezing out from under my eyelashes. I pursed my lips closed and shook my head in refusal. Even though I wasn't getting Ativan, I still wasn't going to take those damn carbamazepine tablets!

My neurosurgeon's nurse practitioner soon appeared on an unscheduled but timely patient visit. Her random stopover was as if God had heard my plea. She fully understood my request and promptly rescued me with an IV Ativan order.

The much-awaited day finally came, and I was rolled into the operating room again. My neurosurgeon lightly anesthetized me with propafol and this time quickly zapped both V2 and V3 nerves with an even higher temperature of 75° C (167° F) of thermal radiant energy. The fiendish torture I had been living with disappeared immediately now that the second rhizotomy had been successfully completed.

Ding, dong ... the wicked witch is dead!

I returned home from the hospital the next day, and for the first time in five months of constant pain and up to four years of periodic "where-the-hell-is-it-coming-from" pain, I was restored to normal. I suddenly had an insane amount of energy. Apparently, my body was trying to compensate for lost time not spent talking on the phone, composing words on my computer, and going out to eat. I was so fired up, I operated at near manic proportion. Because I had barely eaten or drunk anything for eight days and couldn't poop, I needed a good old-fashioned "colon cleansing" to restore my bowels to normal.

Oddly, my body actually had difficulty adjusting to a misery-free lifestyle. I would lie in bed for hours unable to sleep because I was no longer sedated from carbamazepine. I became reacquainted with my old friend, the dirty martini, to help me wind down and relax before bedtime. I haven't used my electric toothbrush in over two years, however, because the vibrations scare me, making me panic with the threat of a return of the nightmarish pain.

Dentists hear complaints of facial pain first

Dental-care professionals play an obvious role in the identification and management of tooth pain. Any tooth deemed responsible must be truly compromised and beyond repair before they perform an extraction. They are cautioned to act conservatively when diagnosing mouth pain.

As E. Sarlani and colleagues write, "The dental practitioner should be familiar with trigeminal neuralgia to avoid unnecessary dental interventions and ensure prompt initiation of appropriate treatment."[4]

Further, according to *Columbia Dental Review*, dental professionals "should be able to formulate an accurate differential diagnosis for facial pain disorders and make the correct decision regarding whether

---

4 E. Sarlani, et al., "Trigeminal Neuralgia in a Patient with Multiple Sclerosis and Chronic Inflammatory Demyelinating Polyneuropathy," *Journal of the American Dental Association* 136 (4): 469–76.

treatment is necessary within their areas of expertise or whether a proper referral is indicated."[5]

Trigeminal neuralgia, like MS, is difficult to diagnose. Since there is no biological marker—no chemical in the blood or urine to indicate the disease—clinicians often rule out conditions that it is not. They will also accumulate a chronology of pain behavior experienced on one side of the face. Although suppressing the pain of TN with anticonvulsants is the most pragmatic beginning approach, surgical treatment with rhizotomy turned out to be a more certain method of eradicating the pain from the damaged nerve.

---

5 A. Rabinovich, J. Fang, and S. Scrivani, "Diagnosis and Management of Trigeminal Neuralgia," *Columbia Dental Review* 5 (2000): 4–7.

Chapter 9
Parenting with MS and Disabilities: Why Not?

When I first found out I had MS, I was afraid I wouldn't be viewed as a "fit parent." The fear of being challenged for the right to rear my children arose from stories I read that characterized people with MS or other disabilities as incompetent for this "physically demanding" job. It was critical that others believed I was up to the task of raising my kids, because I was a single parent and concerned about maintaining the current shared-custody relationship with their father.

I recalled a conversation from 1989: A colleague made a comment about a girl with MS that left a lasting impression. She whispered with disbelief that the day her niece was diagnosed with MS, her husband asked the doctor if she could still have kids. "Can you believe it? With MS?" my colleague asked, shocked that he could even think of such a thing when it was clearly out of the question.

I didn't know anything about MS at the time, but I registered the raw meaning of her words: "People with MS shouldn't have children."

Do disabled people have a right to be parents?

What my colleague said twenty-three years ago reflected the views of our society at the time. Today, although people with disabilities are still subject to stereotyping, parents who are disabled are regarded as capable of giving birth to and raising children. Reasonable adults acknowledge the obligations they have to provide a safe and healthy physical and psychological environment for their children. If a parent satisfies these conditions, are her disabilities relevant?

Unfortunately, there is no law that guarantees parenting rights to a disabled person or assures that he or she will maintain custody of the children. Each parenting case must be addressed individually, and parents who want custody are left to "fight their own fight" and prove their ability to be parents.

When I was diagnosed with MS in early 1999, I knew my role as a parent would be subject to scrutiny. I was a mother of two children, ages five and a half and eight with one father, and a one-year-old with another father. Each father exercised his parenting role and viewed the value of mine in dramatically different ways. The first one was unaccommodating, the second, supportive. The uphill battle to maintain my shared-custody arrangement with the father of my two oldest children turned into the greatest and most unexpected legal challenge I would experience.

First things first: Telling my children I have MS

After my diagnosis, I needed time to digest the life-changing news before I could tell my older children and comfortably introduce potential changes into the family dynamics. Obviously, I had to tell them. I limited the facts to the "here and now" and, to guard against any emotional upsets, I avoided any allusions to an indeterminate future.

Delivering this vague announcement was scary. There was no script or instruction manual to use as a guide. I felt unprepared but pretty certain no one could possibly know the "right" words to say in this situation. I focused on maintaining a reassuring demeanor because, as children do, even at their young ages, my kids easily picked up on such subliminal clues as subtle expressions and tone of voice.

My kids responded better than I expected. My oldest daughter cried and worried that I was going to die. My son wore the face of a brave little man and, being an intellectual, was more interested in the factual information about MS. My one-year-old daughter didn't have a clue. For all three, their biggest concern was whether I would still be able to be their mother. I assured them that MS wouldn't interfere with my ability to be "Mom" but that I wouldn't be as physically active as I had been in the past. My mission now was to honor their trust in me—to be there for them when they needed me, to attend dance recitals, ball games, school programs—to do all the things that moms do.

Telling my children's father about my MS

I was nervous about breaking the news to the father of my oldest two children because he always seemed to find a way to make me feel inadequate as a single parent. He often boasted about his large, happy, stable two-married-adults-who-have-vowed-never-to-be-divorced family; and he was also a stepfather to his wife's three children. I cringed, fearing that he might present my compromised condition as injurious to the children and an opportunity for him to take full custody away from me, leaving me less "parenting jurisdiction."

At that time, disabled parents were slowly being perceived as worthy of caring for their children, but stories of those being denied custodial rights were still common. I worried that skewed traditional beliefs might win, but the idea of *not* raising my children was incomprehensible to me. The liberty to claim rights to your children as a disabled parent wasn't etched in stone. (Thankfully, organizations to support parents with disabilities are becoming more commonplace. An example is the Center for the Rights of Disabled Parents, established in April 2011. Groups like this one didn't exist back then.)

Reluctantly, I phoned my kids' father with the information about my new diagnosis. But instead of gasping with surprise as I had expected, he flippantly claimed to already know about my condition. I immediately realized this was possible, as we had too many friends and family in the medical field with easy access to what is now regarded as confidential health information.

I felt violated and embarrassed that he had prior knowledge of my "secret" health status. But this open exchange of information occurred before the Health Information Privacy and Portability Act (HIPPA), which secures the confidentiality and protection of health data from unauthorized viewing, became law.

I pooh-poohed any inference that my MS would compromise my ability to be an effective mother, but inside I panicked, lacking confidence about how successful I could really be. I had no family nearby and wondered whether I was being fair to my children or hanging on to my parenting role for selfish reasons.

Former homecoming queen with MS loses children

This story of a woman with MS and the relationship with her kids left another indelible impression in my mind. I carpooled with a friend of a friend from Columbus to Lorain, Ohio, in 2000, to attend a wedding shower. During our two-hour drive north, my traveling companion mentioned her plans to stay overnight at her parents' house in her hometown of Wellington, Ohio, only minutes outside of Lorain.

By then, I had had MS for about a year and a half and had read numerous articles about Wellington's reputation of having one of the highest per capita incidences of MS in the United States. My driving companion was curious and intrigued by the eerie MS statistic and the reason for my familiarity with her obscure village.

When I got into her car for our return trip, she couldn't wait to show me a copy of the Sunday edition of the Wellington newspaper. Coincidentally, this special issue of the paper dedicated several pages to a feature on the city's high incidence of MS.

The piece, which detailed the life of a former Wellington High School homecoming queen who developed MS after graduation, featured a nearly five-by-seven-inch photo of her on the front cover. The article described this beautiful girl's life before and after her disability. She appeared stunning in a portrait from her late teen years. After graduation in 1978, she married and had three children. Within fifteen years post-high school, according to the article, "she was stricken by the ravages of MS."

I slowly turned to the next page and looked at pictures of what appeared to be an unkempt woman sitting in an electric wheelchair being spoon-fed. I couldn't help but be shocked that the woman in the wheelchair was the former homecoming queen who had suffered the ruinous consequences of MS. The woman feeding her was her elderly mother, who was visiting her at the nursing home where she resided.

Most perplexing and upsetting was that the ex-husband of the woman with MS gained full custody of their three children and moved several hours south of their Wellington hometown.

There were several coincidences between the Wellington girl's story and my own. I graduated from Lakewood High School the same year, in a suburb of Cleveland located only forty miles away from Wellington. I also lived ten years in another Lake Erie city, Lorain, situated "next door" to her hometown. This attention-grabbing story forced me to examine the life I might anticipate if I had the same debilitating form of MS.

This story also reinforced the message: If you get MS, you're doomed as a parent.

Old-fashioned thinking about MS and parenting

Only two years post-diagnosis, I couldn't muster the strength to lift my feet high enough to walk upstairs. Out of frustration, I called my parents and cried. I'm sure they sensed my overwhelming feeling of defeat regarding my precarious circumstance, because they immediately drove two hours south from Cleveland to Columbus to calm my anxiety.

When my parents finally arrived, I described how surreal it felt to freeze mid-stride and how I had exhausted all my physical and mental effort trying to convince each foot to move my body to the first level of the house, but my feet refused to budge. A major unexpected physical turning point crept up on me that day and caught me unprepared.

My dad listened patiently while I rambled on breathlessly about how scared I was. I couldn't tell whether he was on the same page with me as I shared my frustration, but I knew that he, too, was furious with the dogged way this disease was destroying everything I had become. I understood his anger that MS was ruining the life of the daughter he raised to be so independent.

I anticipated that whatever he said, his words would contain loving advice and support. So, I was stunned to hear him say, "At some point, you know, you're going to have to give up these kids."

Of course, I was thinking, gee, what happened to, "Don't worry, honey. We'll take care of you and the kids"?

My father was a realist and "called a spade, a spade." If he thought I would be unable to take care of myself, why would I think I could care for my children? Realistically, I knew he wouldn't have offered to take the kids, so why was I surprised when he didn't? The logistics with my kids were tricky: my parents lived in Cleveland, and I lived in Columbus with a shared parenting arrangement with my ex-husband, who also lived in Columbus. I guess I just wanted some pity.

My parents were children of old-school thinking in many ways. They were brought up during a time when people who couldn't take care of themselves lived in institutions that could care for them. And they certainly weren't capable of raising children.

For the first time, I recognized that I was on my own, and no one was going to fight this battle for me. Was I fooling myself by believing I could truly take care of my kids? My father's words hit me hard and challenged what little confidence I had.

The shared parenting plan as a disabled parent

My last day of work occurred at the end of 2001. I officially claimed disability from my job as a clinical utilization pharmacist and soon began receiving Social Security disability income.

I had been divorced from the father of my oldest two children for seven years at the time, and because my income was good during that time, I never sought financial assistance to raise our children. But after two years of receiving a meager disability income and observing the increasingly disparate lifestyles my children experienced at each parent's home, I felt the time was right to seek support to help "level the playing field."

To avoid a lengthy and costly trial, we were ordered by the court to iron out our differences and create a new parenting plan under the direction of a mediator, a person licensed to moderate the negotiation process between two adversarial parties. Mediation costs less than involving lawyers and is simpler than resolving a complaint in court, but the process has its weaknesses. The success of the mediation process is largely determined by the strength of the mediator and can allow the stronger-willed party to lead the discussions and ultimately win the argument. In the case of creating a new, shared-parenting plan, my ex-husband found subtle ways to muscle his interests into the final written agreement.

The shared parenting plan contained the directives specifying that if I required a personal caregiver, I would be defined as "unable to parent my children," and full custody would revert to their father.

Both my attorney and the mediator were aware of the language written in the contract, but neither challenged this provision before signing their names. I was too embarrassed and afraid to ask whether the agreement was "fair." In hindsight, I should have sought support for a review of the agreed plan on this topic. No one seemed proficient in the area of domestic disability rights, and I didn't have enough backbone to argue with my ex-husband's objections to parenting while requiring physical assistance. I succumbed to the directives he devised in the parenting contract. I felt powerless to challenge this dubious language. I was in denial that full disability could befall me in the future; and I lost the motivation to fight, stand resolute, and negotiate for adequate financial parenting support in the process.

Three years had passed since the creation of the 2003 shared-parenting plan, and I exercised my right to have an income reevaluation by the Child Support Agency. But instead of complying with the request to provide updated financial information, my oldest two children's father filed a lawsuit for full custodial rights because of my health. Furthermore, he wanted the children's Social Security checks and child support paid to him.

He believed my disabilities from MS were synonymous with an inability to be an adequate parent. His accusations were further diminishing my confidence as I became more reliant on physical assistance. However, I had just met Medicaid eligibility and was entitled to enroll as a "consumer" in the Ohio Home Care Program. I was also working with a team of women caregivers to help me meet my goal of keeping my children.

I couldn't afford legal assistance or find anyone with experience in domestic disability issues, so I composed and filed my own legal papers in my defense. Despite my best efforts, I couldn't locate any legal language or case history that would support me as a disabled parent. I felt hopeless until a good friend discovered and enthusiastically suggested the Ohio Legal Rights Service. Thankfully, I was able to take advantage of their services and a sensible approach to my situation.

Ohio Legal Rights to the rescue

The Ohio Legal Rights Service represents the rights of people with disabilities. The agency provided legal support for civil and employment issues but, unfortunately, not for domestic disputes. One compassionate attorney, however, was touched by my case and felt compelled to fortify my pro se defense (acting as my own attorney) with an amicus brief.

Also known as a "friend of the court" brief, this document was written and filed with the court in support of my parenting as a disabled person. Because neither the person writing the brief nor the entity he represented was a party to the case, the legal rights agency avoided additional court obligations.

The paper emphasized that a disabled parent's ability to raise his or her children existed as long as fundamental parenting standards were met. The amicus brief sent a strong message to the magistrate and judges that my disabilities with MS should not be considered a hindrance to fulfilling my responsibilities as a parent; this ultimately gave me the power to renegotiate my shared-parenting agreement.

The Ohio Legal Rights Service cited a number of legal cases that upheld the rights of handicapped parents. However, I found the following analogy in the amicus brief to be most poignant and memorable:

"Termination of parental rights is the family law equivalent of the death penalty in a criminal case."[1]

I also initiated a request for a guardian ad litem, an attorney who represents the best interests of the children. She met with my kids for an extended period of time to better understand their areas of concern with both parents. She also arranged individual meetings with their father and me to get to the heart of any concerns we might have.

After numerous continuances and rescheduled trial dates, our case was needlessly dragged out until it became a grueling five-year debacle. Since I continued to be an effective parent despite having caregivers attending to me, the whole "unfit parent" issue became irrelevant. I was able to continue the fifty-fifty shared-parenting agreement with my ex-husband and the long-standing relationship with my kids until high school graduation.

Another parallel disabled parenting case?

"Quadriplegic Mother May Lose Custody of Son" was the title of a *New York Times* article dated January 4, 2010, in the Internet publication *Shine,* on Yahoo! I was involved with my own custody litigation during that time; and, since I can be a bit superstitious, I avoided checking the status of the court's decision on this particular case. I was afraid to discover that custody had been awarded to the "able-bodied" father.

The article described a girl named Kaney O'Neill, a former navy airman apprentice, who severed her spinal cord after the wind blew her off a balcony during Hurricane Floyd in 1999. From this dramatic event, she had no use of her legs and minimal use of her arms. She became pregnant nine years later and prepared for the birth of her baby by recruiting her family, a regular caregiver, and a service dog. Nonetheless, she still had to fight criticism that she was unable to be an adequate mother to her child.

Her ex-boyfriend filed a lawsuit for full custody of their son. Kaney O'Neill described this as the toughest battle she ever had to

---

1 *Smith vs. Smith*, 77 Ohio App. 3d. 1, 16 (1991)

face. The father charged that she was "not a fit and proper parent" and that her disability "greatly limited her ability to care for the minor or even wake up if the minor is distressed." In May 2011, Kaney O'Neill *won* the lawsuit.

What is the definition of a good parent?

Courts have been unable to agree on the definition of a "fit and proper" parent. The California Supreme Court set a precedent in 1979, clarifying that the "essence of parenting is not to be found in the harried rounds of daily carpooling" but rather "in the ethical, emotional, and intellectual guidance the parent gives the child throughout his formative years." A parent's disability cannot be the sole basis upon which custody is denied.[2]

Outside of the courts, the definition of a good parent varies, but there are more similarities than differences. Examples include being available to shoulder tears and jubilation; listen attentively; eat together; help children manage little struggles, such as homework and relationships; boost their confidence; prepare them for successful lives; and defend them or "have their back" when appropriate. Other interpretations encompass expressing love and affection; listening to them; making them feel safe; praising them; avoiding criticism and focusing on the behavior; being consistent; spending time with each child individually; being a role model; and letting them experience life for themselves without losing control.

Was I living up to the definition of a "good" parent who was able to meet the challenges of parenting? Could I fulfill my role as a mother while I was disabled and in a wheelchair? These were the questions I asked myself.

Who can be a parent?

Is an adult who relies on a nanny to nurture her children still a good parent? How about an adult who always stays late at work, travels for

---

2 Marriage of Carney, 24 Cal. 3d 725, 598 P.2d 472—[Cal. Sup. Ct. 1979]

long periods of time, or is away from home day after day? On the other hand, what about the stepparent who feeds and transports the children and does their laundry in order to allow the biological parent time to meet his or her professional and personal goals? Is the biological parent acting as a fit parent in this case? What if the biological parent has a problem with chemical abuse or spends hours sitting in front of a television?

If these are acceptable "absentee" behaviors on the part of able-bodied parents, why then is there concern that a person with a disability would do any worse? Disabled parents run the spectrum between good and bad, just as able-bodied individuals do; but, unfortunately, some able-bodied parents see their roles as parents as an entitlement rather than a privilege or an earned position.

My kids after fourteen years with my MS

I miss not being physically involved with my kids. I like to horse around, dance, ride bikes, and cut hair. I wish I could cook with my son and put fingernail polish and makeup on my girls. Now that my son and youngest daughter play guitar, I wish I could strum along with them and learn contemporary music from them.

I continue to stay focused on doing things I can do and cling to the notion that my children are learning character-building lessons of great value from me through the things I do with them; say to them; and, most important, the things they watch me do for myself.

My children are twenty-two, nineteen, and fifteen; and I'm proud to say that each is self-assured and fiercely independent. Most of their lives have been under the care of a disabled mother, and they know I have willfully provided them with as much love and support as I could give.

My youngest daughter has only known me as disabled and, out of the three children, has handled me with the greatest of ease. Since birth, she grew up accustomed to being reared by a mother in a wheelchair. I strongly credit her father and his family for the way she interacts with me because she has only seen them treat me as "normal."

Nonetheless, my children have probably become more self-sufficient than other children their age because of the time they have spent living with me. They took care of the little things by themselves— throwing together some pasta, borrowing an egg from a neighbor, washing a few clothes, making a snack tray, cleaning and dressing a boo-boo on a leg, and the list goes on. The oldest two are in college, extremely resourceful and demonstrating that they are capable of fearless behavior. They are compassionate human beings who express deep concern for those in need and do not unnecessarily worry about my health.

Evidence of increased acceptance of disabled parents

The positive way in which society views disabled parents is gaining momentum. Disabled parents are reaching out to admit they need assistance with accomplishing everyday tasks and getting the help they need to be competent parents.

In the same January 4, 2010, *New York Times* article, "Should a Quadriplegic Mom Have Custody?" I refer to above, Anne Armstrong of Illinois, an occupational therapist since 1986, was quoted as saying, "We didn't see as many parents with disabilities even a decade ago, but the taboo is definitely fading. I see a lot of self-advocacy on the part of these parents. They know how to ask for help and use the resources."

My advice for parenting with MS and disabilities

Parents with MS and disabilities need to be creative in compensating for their weaknesses. Because I was unable to get around effectively and comfortably, I found that I spoke to my children with greater eye contact and more sincerity, and I listened to them more intently.

In some strange, unimaginable way, the emotional and intellectual bonds with each of my kids were strengthened. I bolstered the tone of my voice and reinforced my involvement with their interests to further improve our connection with each other. Whether I could or couldn't drive myself, I still focused on booking the same types of outings. I visited parks and festivals and went on shopping excursions.

I have gone to a sizable number of rock concerts, theater productions, musicals, and a different Cirque du Soleil production with each of my children.

Over the years, each child adapted and developed a unique relationship with me and my wheelchair. My son liked to push the manual and run like a rickshaw driver. My girls mastered the manipulation of the sensitive controls to drive the electric model. They would bicker over the number of times and duration each would sit on my lap and freely navigate the territory.

My kids know that dignity is one of my priorities. When my bedroom door is shut, I am with a healthcare aide. They all recognize when "private Mommy time" must be honored. This separation of Mommy as a disciplinarian from seeing Mommy's bare bottom has perpetuated the parental status I wished to maintain. They also get involved with a lot of my needs that aren't quite so intimate: getting the hair out of my mouth or off my forehand, giving me a sip of a drink, wiping my nose, stirring a pot, and cleaning their "damn" rooms. (My loving children complete household tasks with the same enthusiasm and dedication as any able-bodied parent's children do. This simply means that, just like any kids, *most* of the time they cooperate, and *sometimes* their lives "need to be threatened" in order to get them to accomplish anything asked of them.)

My children play, converse, laugh, share popular music, and use the same jargon as their peers, even though they have a mother who can't physically participate as most can. I can't take part in the Parent-Teacher Organization (PTO), transportation, hands-on activities, parties (most homes are not accessible), or my son's high school football games. But hopefully I have explained right from wrong, scolded, praised, told valuable stories, and gotten them to laugh at a few dumb jokes. They seem to be more emotionally resilient, independent, and conversant with adults. It is my hope that they will evolve into compassionate, understanding, and patient people as a result of their experience with me.

Chapter 10
Depression, Loneliness, and Fear: Upstream Without a Paddle

"No one knows what it's like to be the sad man ... behind blue eyes."
—The Who

There's no question about it. Having a disease like MS is scary as hell. Think about it: unexplained erosion in the brain and spinal cord and corrupting messages sent to a chance destination anywhere throughout the vast, far-reaching neurological frontier.

"Houston, we have a problem."

And, yes, these damages produce unexpected interruptions to normal bodily performance. The unpredictable dysfunctions can be irritating, embarrassing, and frightening. One becomes a prisoner in her own body. There is no escaping the resulting effect on the psyche.

Just the mere thought of having MS made me sad, as if a perfect stranger just punched me in the stomach, ran away, and left me to ache in confusion. Anyone can understand that feeling a little bummed out would be a natural reaction. But if "the blues" stick around too long, as they did with me, counseling and an antidepressant may be necessary. Depression.

It seemed to me that the friends I used to see didn't come around as much anymore or just disappeared. People naturally avoid heartbreak and being around a transparent, cheerless heart. I found it easy to slip into isolation, like an injured animal that disappears to lick its wounds in the forest. Loneliness.

My body defiantly continued to operate on its own terms. Obligations and responsibilities still awaited in my world; there was so much I needed to do and so much I wanted to do. Now what? How long will this go on? Will this uncontrollable fiend ever disappear? How can I function at work? Manage family activities? I wanted so badly to be a "normal" human again. Fear.

MS is a forever disease. You have no choice but to adjust and coexist with it. Life goes on "as scheduled." Within four years of my diagnosis I went through everything at the top of the list of stressors: I divorced my first husband, began a doctorate program, remarried, withdrew from college, had a baby, was *diagnosed with MS*, got divorced *again*, relocated home and office from a multilevel home to a ranch, "retired" from work, and applied for disability income . . . and I was just getting started. I didn't know if I was coming or going; I wrote the playbook as I went.

Depression, loneliness, fear. These three sullen emotions made up for all the physical MS pain I was fortunate enough to avoid (*except* from trigeminal neuralgia). These morose feelings never appeared in any stepwise order but ran together intertwined.

My first notable post-diagnosis reaction

I stood by and watched the energetic opening dance scene of an Austin Powers movie on TV the day after my diagnosis. Mike Myers's characters are typically a hoot, but this time I wasn't laughing. I was distracted by sound and movement, not comedy. Although I hadn't ever danced like that before, I just realized that even if I wanted to, I would never be able to. Ever.

How do others feel with MS?

"Is there anybody out there?" —Pink Floyd

They say "misery loves company." It must be true because I really wanted to connect with others who were dealing with MS. I wanted to know how they made it work in their lives. Through my search I found two main categories of support groups: those online and those in my local area.

Online MS help groups

Voyeuristically, I peered into chat rooms and weblogs at different

Internet sites that provided a forum for people with MS. I visited WebMD, Copaxone.com, Avonex.com, AcceleratedCure.com, and anywhere else my search engine would take me. Most of these dedicated MS sites were pretty much alike. They differed only by the mix of those who created them—the individuals who participated and often contributed their stories and suggestions. I found AcceleratedCure.com to be the most informative, as it included national stories and research updates, but each was helpful in its own way.

Local MS support groups

I wanted to meet some real, live people with MS, so I attended a local National Multiple Sclerosis Society group meeting held at a church in Columbus. I chose this one because the speaker was presenting on a nutritional topic. Bracing the weight of my body with a cane in my right hand, I wobbled into a room full of thirty to forty attendees. I thought I would see a bunch of people using assistive walking devices, but only two others actually brought canes, which were never used and remained propped up behind their chairs for the evening. One middle-aged woman actually drove in on a motorized scooter but transferred herself into a folding chair before the program started.

After the meeting, I hung around a small group that gathered to commiserate about different MS issues—constipation, urinary hesitancy, and fatigue. One woman announced she was legally blind and unable to drive. Fortunately, her husband could drive her around town. None of these people fought the same physical demons as I did.

I hadn't been diagnosed long and believed I had a lot to learn about MS. I was paranoid that others might wonder what I may or may not be doing to be in such poor physical condition. Since no one else seemed to have concerns similar to mine, I felt justified in not attending this same group again.

Later, when it became apparent primary-progressive MS was my full diagnosis, I couldn't locate a specific support group. Were others like me reluctant to venture out of their homes, or did they lack the ability and/or transportation to do so?

As I continued my search for people who could relate to what I was going through, I was put in touch with a fellow my age who also had PPMS. He "retired" from a well-paying job in information technology; and, from what I understood from the woman who connected us, he was quite a looker and player. He and I communicated well on an intellectual level and were also candid about how MS had ruined our social lives.

At the end of our first phone conversation, he said, "What I miss most is waking up next to a woman's naked body." I was thrown off a bit by his comment because I was embarrassed that some guy I barely knew was talking to me so openly. I wondered, "Will this happen to me?"

I understood what he meant about sex being what he missed most. I was recently divorced (a second time and definitely not interested in a third marriage); but I, too, missed this intimacy and the freedom to be like Inga from the movie Young Frankenstein, "Roll, Roll, Roll in Zee Hay." Of course, it wasn't the word *sex* that he used to describe this animalistic pleasure, but for all intents and purposes, it's the same thing. Conversations with him gave MS a human face. Technical details and clinical terms can be found in plenty of sources, but in order to understand a real MS experience, it's far more valuable to listen to someone who can describe real-life, firsthand encounters with the disease.

The dancer with MS

On another blog I spotted comments by a woman who was distraught over the loss of her ability to dance. She was a thirty-five-year-old professional dancer who depended on her agility to perform well for her livelihood. She also equated her attractiveness with moving her body seductively. Her body's new limitations caused her anguish, and she sought the support of others with MS who felt the disease had robbed them of their sensuality. The dancer's grief was understandable; I felt the same way when I was losing my feminine poise. Although our circumstances were different, making even an indirect connection made us both feel better, somehow.

Losses from MS

The real sadness of MS is the consequence of the precious things it destroys in our lives that may not be immediately identified as "conventional losses." Loss of loved ones due to death or divorce is a frequently addressed heartache, but sadly, the grief of a disabling condition is not. Loss of a pet or even facing an "empty nest" when children leave home are topics with which others can empathize, but sorrow from the things MS shatters is not. Yet, these losses are as deeply felt and as hurtful. To better express the terrible real-life impact of such losses, I share the following examples of loss of independence, physical functioning, identity, and self-image.

Loss of independence

You don't realize how often you flick, smooth, and tousle your hair in a five-minute period. How many times do you push hair away from your face or scratch your nose? If you can't do it yourself, every time you need one of these tasks done for you, you must interrupt someone's activity to take care of this minuscule task. You could have dozens of these requests within an hour's time, so you learn to prioritize your concerns and only call for help when you are desperate.

Since I can't style my own hair and apply my own makeup, I'm almost always unhappy with the way I look, no matter who primped me. The part in my hair could be a millimeter off from the way I like it, but because I am not able to craft it myself, I'm frustrated and miserable.

I remind myself that some desires are unreasonable. Once, when I was a hairstylist-to-be in cosmetology school, an older woman handed me a picture of Victoria Principal, a beautiful actress from TV series *Dallas* in the late 1970s and '80s, and asked me to make her hairstyle look like Victoria Principal's in the photo. I know my personal expectations may be as unrealistic as hers were; yet, I still hold a passive narcissistic desire to be beautiful.

Another difficult part of disability is the loss of anonymity—no private time and no privacy. Someone must always be with me to help with just about everything. But even if I had enough money for a modified house with high-tech electronic gadgetry everywhere around me, while it would buy me greater independence, there isn't any mechanical solution for wiping away a stray hair, a bug, or piece of fuzz from my face.

Loss of function

"I've seen a lot (from war), but there ain't nothing like the sight of an amputated spirit. There is no prosthetic for that."

—Retired Army Ranger Lt. Col. Frank Slade, *Scent of a Woman*

The loss of *function* is intensely wounding. I know what it's like to anguish over losing an active life. MS strips you of all those things that you can no longer do or be.

On one occasion, I remember rushing at the last minute, to assemble a hot dish for a potluck at my daughter's preschool. As I prepared the dish for travel, I lost my balance, and in an attempt to prevent falling to the floor, I braced my left hand against the burning, flat porcelain surface of the stove. The searing heat literally melted the skin off from the bottom of my thumb to my wrist, and a large fluid-filled blister grew in its place.

But it wasn't only when I was rushing about that I hurt myself. Whenever I transferred back and forth from the wheelchair to the toilet, my legs always seemed to get in the way. The skin on my calves, shins, and ankles became snagged, scraped, or poked by the chair's jagged, bolted edges.

A friend was coming to terms with a severe car crash injury that left her unable to play competitive softball. I can relate to the loss of a skill that gave me enjoyment but that I no longer have. I was a skilled hairstylist and had a reputation as the family "barber." I was disappointed when my hands and fingers began to lose their ability to hold hair in my left hand and cut it adeptly with my right.

Loss of self-image and identity

Closely tied to the loss of function and independence is the loss of self-image. Self-image is how you perceive yourself. Identity, according to the *Merriam-Webster* dictionary, is the "distinguishing character or personality of an individual." Although seemingly not as significant as functional losses, losing this self-perception can be damaging to one's sense of value and internalized as a form of grief.

The girl from Ipanema?

I took pride in my tall, thin, five-foot-seven-inch stature. I was never a model and don't have an athletic body, but I could carry my frame well enough that it wouldn't hurt anyone's eyes to look at it. Now, I sit in a wheelchair and am three and a half feet tall. I have long fingers, and my nails were always presentable. My nail beds were deep, long, and attractive, thanks to my Spanish roots. My nails were always long enough for a good back scratching; but now you never see them, because with my fingers permanently contracted, they are buried in the palms of my hands. Even Botox injections didn't relax them enough to lie as flat on my lap as I would have liked.

My thin form is also gone. Although my stomach was never washboard flat, I was conscious of when useless fatty curves appeared on my abdomen. A dozen or two sit-ups would typically remedy little bumps. After about four years of losing trunk strength, however, I began to lose firmness in my abdominal muscles. Although I hadn't gained more than a few pounds, my midline spread out without definition. I compare my body shape with the evil and fat slothlike character Jabba the Hut of *Star Wars* or the animated little green mucus people in the Mucinex commercials.

The day following Michael Jackson's death, I overheard an interview with physician and author Deepak Chopra. He spoke of his twenty-year friendship with Michael and recalled that Michael Jackson, arguably one of the most outstanding musical performers who ever lived, was depressed by several "demons," one of which was his poorly misunderstood battle with loss of skin color from vitiligo.[1]

---

1 Vitiligo is mentioned as an autoimmune disease by Dr. Chopra and that "stress may be a

All the money in the world could not replace the pigment in his skin, which contributed to the image he had of himself, or the peace of mind and happiness it brought him.

A fall from grace?

In the fall of 2010, David Cassidy, of *Partridge Family* fame, appeared on Donald Trump's reality show *The Celebrity Apprentice*. Cassidy was a wildly popular teen idol in the 1970s. Now, more than forty years had passed since his heyday as an international sensation who left so many teenage girls starstruck.

When Cassidy participated as a contestant on *The Celebrity Apprentice*, his "finish" was disappointing as he no longer came across as "every girl's dream" and was noticeably outshined by the younger male contestants on the show. His demeanor was reserved and a bit uncomfortable.

I wondered what it must feel like inside David Cassidy's skin at that moment. Did he mourn the loss of the iconic it-boy image he once had? I'm not a celebrity, but I think I can understand the loss of those things that define them—youth, good looks, popularity. I get it.

What do you *do*?

If you have always defined yourself by what you "do"—your career, job, or achievements—you limit your redefinition if you want to include only those things you formerly did. Find new activities you *can* do to redefine yourself. This doesn't mean that your old self has to be discarded. What makes you "you" still remains, despite whatever functions you have lost. Although I still dabble with my pharmacy knowledge in different capacities, I am trying to increase my knowledge in the area of writing and publishing, thus changing the way I define myself.

(causative) factor." "Stress was a problem in Michael's childhood." *Countdown with Keith Olbermann,* MSNBC, June 27, 2008.

Proud to be a pharmacist

I am a pharmacist. I worked most of my life as a pharmacist and still live and think like one. Pharmacy had always played a huge role in my life's satisfaction and was rewarding intellectually, academically, and financially. I also had serious intentions of getting a doctorate degree in the field and have maintained an active pharmacy license year after year, although my professional involvement is limited to assisting friends or family with medication management.

What kind of car do you drive?

I owned a pearl-colored Lexus 400 LS that drove as smoothly as flying a jet on a clear day. I loved that car, the feel of driving it, the prestige of owning it, and the symbol of professional achievement it conveyed.

As my MS progressed, I needed this pristine car to be equipped with garish-looking hand controls. As time passed, I had to accommodate for my other functional losses, as well. My legs grew weaker and so did my ability to climb in and out of the driver's seat. I began to understand the helpless feeling of motor-function losses and needed to change more things in my driving environment. And yes, that meant getting rid of my beloved Lexus and replacing it with a vehicle that worked better with my disabilities.

While awaiting delivery of a custom-built scooter for use outside my home, I needed a vehicle that could transport it easily from place to place. There was nothing stylish about a minivan, but I knew it would suit my need to haul my three-wheeled mobile device. I reluctantly purchased a wheelchair-accessible Dodge Grand Caravan minivan with a foldout ramp.

From the luxurious and emotional high of driving a Lexus to a frumpy, gutted-out, wheelchair-accessable van with a lowered floor, I was reduced to a sexless life in a sexless vehicle with an underside that dragged on the surface of every slightly elevated spot on the road.

Loss of social involvement

When I didn't have MS, I considered myself quite social. I always kept my social calendar busy with parties, visits, and entertaining events. I enjoyed hosting get-togethers, as well as attending them. When I first became disabled, I was still focused on staying active in all types of community events, but within a dozen years, I began to change my attitude about remaining involved.

I didn't like the disenfranchised way I felt with some able-bodied guests at parties. I hated it when I ran into people I had not seen for some time. I often felt patronized. "How *are* you?" "How are you *feeling*?" Or the one that always kills me, "But you *look* so good!"

I don't like attending social gatherings where people are standing up the entire time. Unless it's a dinner party where people are comfortably sitting, they are standing in their dress garb, neatly appointed from head to toe, with women often in three-inch heels. If you are in a wheelchair, you are at a huge disadvantage because people can't hear you or see your lips move. Those on their feet have little idea that you are incredibly put out and very uncomfortable.

I can't visit most friends' homes that have multiple floors. One friend has a cobblestone entrance, and others have narrow doorways. Shopping at unique secondhand stores and boutiques is nearly impossible because of narrow spacing between clothing and precariously placed items on unstable shelving.

Attending movies requires me to sit in a special spot, typically in the first three rows of the theater. Who in her right mind would voluntarily choose to sit so close to the big screen where the cinema images are magnified to such a degree that the pictures are nearly unrecognizable?

Socializing with former colleagues and friends became less frequent over time because I began to feel an overwhelming concern about the presence of my wheelchair. Could I get into the building? Fit through the door? Would enough strong people be available and willing to propel me up an angle? And sometimes I'd think, "I'm sick of being such a pain in the ass."

Physical encumbrances and hindrances dampened relationships with friends because it seemed everything I did with them involved less spontaneity and more preplanning. But was it really physical setbacks that prevented me from participating as fully as I once did? Probably not. I think what had the most negative impact on my full participation in activities I used to enjoy was more *psychological* than *physical.*

My inability to feel at ease in a social setting is not always because I can't get through the doors or don't like what I'm wearing. The reason is that no one is looking at me at eye level. I absolutely hate the idea of people looking over me as if I were invisible. How difficult it must be to be a little person!

Fears—usual and customary for MS sufferers

Chances are, the questions those of us with MS have are universal.

What could I look forward to? I felt trapped and unable to accomplish anything worthwhile. I feared the uncertainty of how I was going to manage this menacing disease, my unknown future, and raising my three children. I worried about whether I was strong enough to endure what was certain to be an uphill battle.

Tough but natural questions with MS

"Will I look disheveled and sickly?"

"How will I get around town? Can I still travel?"

"Will I need a wheelchair?"

"Who will take care of me if I can't take care of myself?"

"How bad will my condition get?"

"How will my savings, relationships, independence be affected?"

"How will I handle a life with MS?"

Conclusion

Okay. Rant over. On the brighter side (there really *is* a brighter side)—most people with MS don't end up in a wheelchair (using one is easier than struggling to walk without one … just saying…)

Plus, if I want to go places and do things, the list of where I can visit and activities I can engage in is vast. Today, the Americans with

Disabilities Act (ADA) has opened the world, or much of it, to people with disabilities by making physical accommodations available. ADA standards have been applied to sidewalk curbs, commercial buildings, and public transportation. To comply with the law, business and government establishments must be "handicapped accessible." ADA has made it so that individuals with disabilities are afforded the same opportunities as the general population to participate in cultural and social activities.

Typically, the only thing holding me back is me. If I have all the necessary accommodations for my body's limitations, I realize the answer lies in my attitude.

"The only thing greater than fear is hope."
  —Suzanne Collins, author of *The Hunger Games*

Chapter 11
Attitude Is Everything

Tough times don't last, but tough people do.

Agood attitude prevails over a bad one. We know this truth, but what makes for a good attitude? How do you get one? Put a shiny smile on your face and say pleasantries? Not if *you* don't believe what's on your face or what comes out of your mouth. Attitude is a sincere expression that emerges from deep within your human core.

My body froze like a deer in the headlights when the doctor voiced his conclusion. The words he spoke were dumbfounding. I gave off a laissez-faire attitude about the news and turned up my nose as if to say, "MS? Oh yeah; I knew that." It may have taken a few years after I was diagnosed to realize that, with MS, I could either live with it or stop living.

Some feel defeated by a life with MS and can't adjust to the new circumstance. This negativity creates a bad attitude, which drains energy, deteriorates the soul, and brings on depression, poor health, ruinous relationships, and risk of suicide. A good attitude, on the other hand, attracts positive outcomes—creativity, happiness, likability, success, perseverance, and energy—as well as preventing the above-mentioned damaging consequences.

The choice of outlook was pretty clear. My internal preference is to be happy, but I still do believe in a "good, healthy cry." (I don't think this expression of sadness should be denied; it may be the best first step at dealing with a distressing reality.) So, I celebrated in a few "pity parties" but committed to limiting the amount of time I felt sorry for myself. Then, I moved on and didn't look back.

I stayed open-minded and tried a number of methods to control this animal called MS. The disease, however, became "boss" and imposed limitations on what I could and could not do. Life with MS became crazy tough … but doable.

When will I be "my old self" again?

When I was first diagnosed, friends and family tried to quell my apprehensions about MS by assuring me that researchers were optimistic about the outlook.

"You just wait. In five or ten years, there will be a cure for MS. Science is moving so fast." I wanted so badly to believe this was true that it was only natural for me to keep my hope alive for redemption from this disease.

By 2006, seven years had passed since my diagnosis, and still no MS treatment was on the horizon. I spent hours on the Internet searching for a promising restoration to health. Day after day, with no up-and-coming "cure" for this neurological nightmare in sight, I realized that holding my breath was in vain. I lost interest in monitoring for scientific breakthroughs. I had to get used to it and start making lemonade from these lemons.

Believe me, I was despondent about the grim news. My body was a prisoner to MS, and I hated what it was doing to me physically. Once I began to come to terms with my new physical existence, I knew that turning back the clock was not something I could do. It was time for my new reality and optimism to walk hand-in-hand, peacefully. Yeah, I could deal with this.

Explaining to a stranger why even bad situations can be a good thing

To be clear, I have no degree in or have ever researched the power of the mind. My psychology training is limited to one college course my freshman year at The Ohio State University. Next, scientific writing is the only type of composition I've ever known. It's straightforward, "cut and dried." Facts, numbers, figures, incidents, and frequencies are concrete and understandable. Numbers are precise and quantitative, but describing feelings is vague—nebulous and qualitative.

Yet, I knew an upbeat outlook was vital. The mere act of convincing myself to be content counterbalanced the toxic nature of feeling deprived by a life with MS. The phrase, "Fake it till you make it" became my mantra for a time.

An optimistic perspective should be an inherent part of everyone's internal operating system, just as the human core temperature is about 98.6° F. I viewed myself as disassembled, deficient, and useless in the beginning; but eventually found some desirable, workable characteristics that I had never tapped into. I learned to identify the positives in a negative situation and "think outside the box." (Example: Handicap seats often provide better viewing than general seating.)

I was deeply moved by the movie *The Diving Bell and the Butterfly*, based on the book by Jean Dominique Bauby, the former editor in chief of *Elle* magazine, France. Jean Dominique had a major stroke at forty-two years old, leaving him in a condition known as "locked-in syndrome." With the only remaining movement limited to the muscles that controlled his left eyeball and eyelid, he "dictated" an entire book by blinking for each letter of the words used to share his very unusual experience. I could identify with so much of his physical incapacitation. Jean Dominique and I were both paralyzed in our forties; had a dry, sarcastic brand of humor; and believed we had gained far more than what we lost.

"Had I been blind and deaf? Or did it take the white light of disaster to find my true nature?"
—Jean Dominique Bauby

Capitalize on other strengths
A dreadful disease like MS is not needed to realize you have promising but dormant skills to be illuminated. How exciting to uncover and showcase valuable features that have simply been overlooked!

Humans have a profound capacity to compensate for losses. In my case, my mental acuity has increased as my physical activity has declined.

I was intrigued by the title of a book called *Success from Failure: The Paradox of Design,* by Henry Petroski. Apparently, Petroski focuses on innovations inspired by faux pas in manufacturing history. He illustrates that setbacks teach us more than triumphs and that success breeds catastrophe unlike failure, which nurtures insight. I believe opportunities to *reengineer with improvements* can occur on a personal basis, as well. Notice the number of entrepreneurial businesses that increase when the economy is poor.

Keep your sanity. Stay busy.

I became fatigued and dozed off easily during the day, anytime, anywhere. Subconsciously, I must have hoped I would wake up from a power nap and be back to "normal." I needed to stop holding my breath, waiting to be rejuvenated from a lull, and improve my quality of life. My brain was floating in a zero-gravity environment, and I needed to draw myself to the surface of my planet and get going.

"Staying busy" has a broad definition. I see it as innovating ways to spend your time and energy meaningfully. Keeping myself occupied serves two purposes: it utilizes my resources productively and alleviates wasted energy spent thinking about myself and my hopeless health condition.

I missed working in my clinical pharmacy profession and resurrected my skills to offer medication-management services to senior adults. I also became comfortable wearing a microphone headband and operating my voice-recognition software and later the infrared mouse to control the cursor on my computer screen. I composed business documents, correspondence, and personal manuscripts. I wrote … and wrote … and wrote … and wrote.

When I tired of wordsmithing, the easiest and most enjoyable remedy for occupying my mind was to play the game of computer

Scrabble. I downloaded this singular competition first as a distraction, but the game quickly became an addiction and a healthy diversion from sulking. I spent hours playing this game, challenging myself mentally and improving my vocabulary.

Even unpleasant events became a distraction from my MS. Over a five-year stretch of time, I was mired in several legal and life calamities—an eighteen-month criminal case against a thieving caregiver, a five-year child custody litigation (described in Chapter 9 on parenting with MS), the death of my father due to bladder cancer, my own bladder cancer, and the indescribable pain of trigeminal neuralgia.

In 2011, I began writing this book about my successes, failures, and eye-opening experiences with MS, hoping that those who read my story might benefit. The long journey has been a healthy exercise that keeps me looking forward instead of focusing solely on my illness or dwelling on a past that will never return.

Metaphorically speaking, you need to install a set of antilock brakes to weather the slippery roads of an uncertain diagnosis and regain your traction and composure. People with the ability to keep their alignment on rocky roads seem to share the common denominator of a positive attitude. And while not seeking a sunnier approach to living may be the path of least resistance, why choose that route? Such negativity leads to a lousy existence.

Some people hang on to their negative attitudes with the stubbornness of a child. For instance, once I tried to coach my older daughter to disregard the taunting stares and attempts at psychological sabotage by her younger sister. She was unable to muster the emotionless facial expression to nonchalantly ignore her; so, she lost because she was incapable of changing her tactics. It's tough to alter a mind-set.

I focus on self-empowerment. I avoid physical activities I can't do and, instead, concentrate on improving my mental performance. I will never dance, or ice skate again; but I must have been put in a position to serve those around me in some significant way. I dedicate more time to my kids, read constantly, and try to write about my life in a meaningful way. I want to know how I can be of benefit to the world around me in ways I may have overlooked in the past.

The power of confidence

My early knowledge that I had MS disassembled my life. Until then, I thought I had everything under control, but suddenly I felt helpless and didn't know how to piece my life back together. One day, at an athletic shoe store with my kids, I stared at a large, five-foot Nike poster. It pictured a woman running on a dark, wet, deserted road wearing a determined face and covered in sweat. At the bottom of the poster was the world-renowned slogan, "Just Do It." I never was a runner, but this inspirational motto was incredibly timely.

I have restarted an active lifestyle—going out to restaurants, shopping, and seeing friends. I have ventured away from the confines of my home and into the world around me in order to stimulate my mind. Staying active draws me out of isolation and fortifies my confidence.

How do others deal with MS?

In the preceding chapter, I described how I sought to discover how other people *felt* with MS, but I knew that was plain commiserating, a powwow of complaints and moans. My emphasis should have been on how others *were dealing with* MS. There are all sorts of blogs and websites full of people with MS sharing their woes, concerns, and hopes for salvation. After a lot of digging around, asking questions, and plenty of dead-end roads, I was able to develop *solutions*.

Where does God fit in with attitude?

I believe in God as my "higher power," but I'm not sure if I should credit my positive attitude to religious inspiration. I asked one of my personal-care aides, a devout Jehovah's Witness, what the Bible says regarding the power of attitude. She cited the following reference:

"For when I am weak, then I am powerful." *2 Corinthians 12:7–10*

She explained that Paul, one of Jesus Christ's apostles, was being stoned, and in his darkest hour, he felt his greatest power emerge at a time of his greatest weakness. As Paul underwent provocation, he professed that where he fell short, God would supply the deficit. The Bible elaborates that the greater the deficit, the more power Paul would receive from God.

This phrase was posted in my office for months, and those who read it were curious about the meaning. How can you possibly be weak and powerful at the same time? I understand what this scripture means, not because I am somehow "holy" enough to be worthy of divine comprehension, but because I live it. A secular interpretation of this statement would be "You're stronger than you think you are." Believe it. You are.

The power of hope

"We must accept finite disappointment, but never lose infinite hope."
—Martin Luther King Jr.

Reading the online edition of *Psychology Today* one afternoon, I came across the blog, "Intense Emotions and Strong Feelings," by Mary C. Lamia. Lamia writes, "Hope structures your life in anticipation of the future and influences how you feel in the present ... The positive feelings you experience as you look ahead, imagining ... who you are going to be, can alter how you currently view yourself."

She goes on to make this most poignant observation:

"Having hope is to imagine a positive outcome ...

Faith that things will be better is a positive driver." [1]

An outstanding example of the power of hope is a clinical drug trial. Every new medication the Food and Drug Administration (FDA) reviews for market approval must be compared to a placebo pill. Although a placebo has no active ingredient, it has the power to evoke a suggested effect and can produce a physiological response similar to the therapeutic effect of the active drug. Therefore, the study

---

1 M. C. Lamia, "The Power of Hope, and Recognizing When It's Hopeless," Intense Emotions and Strong Feelings (blog), *Psychology Today*, June 29, 2011; http://www.psychologytoday.com/blog/intense-emotions-and-strong-feelings/201106/the-power-hope-and-recognizing-when-its-hopeless.

results must show a meaningful (statistically significant) difference between the results generated by the active drug and those generated by the placebo.

This placebo effect tells us that to some extent, our beliefs and hopes can translate into physiological changes. Although being realistic is important so that we aren't constantly having our hopes dashed, staying positive has real health benefits that shouldn't be underestimated.

Fear begets a negative attitude; knowledge begets a positive one

No question about it, being diagnosed with a potentially debilitating disease is frightening. Losing control of your bodily functions is unsettling, and not knowing what other symptoms may await you is daunting. Fear-driven anxiety can create a dreadful attitude.

Educating yourself is key to fighting back this anxiety. If you know what you can do to compensate for losses caused by MS, your self-assurance and confidence will increase. Being aware of your options to improve functioning will help calm your fears. When you know what you are facing, you are better equipped to take control of your health care, and that empowerment alone can bring about a more positive attitude.

Humor is the best medicine; lighten up and laugh

Allow yourself to laugh. Laughter is great medicine that produces many positive physiological effects. Studies have shown that laughter can reduce stress, decrease the experience of pain, and increase immunity. Laughter is pleasurable and amusing.

Beyond intelligence and common sense, I think the most important survival trait is a good sense of humor. I don't take myself too seriously and can laugh at myself. I allow myself some leeway, a margin of error, and make sure it's okay to fumble. If I didn't, I would be certain to disappoint myself often.

My sense of humor keeps me amused (even when no one else thinks I'm funny). Laughter is my saving grace and has brought me through the most troubling times. It is also my remedy for grief. A good laugh is critically important to my emotional health and physical well-being. Laughing exercises my chest muscles, makes my breathing stronger, rescues me from the wrath of depression, and is a valuable commodity for dissolving hurtful situations. Hilarity, especially, protects my sanity.

Wearing a sincere smile on my face also has benefits. It creates peace of mind, brings the benefit of joy, reduces facial wrinkles, and can turn an acidic situation into one more digestible. A good sense of humor translates into a good attitude.

Sense-of-humor inspiration

"If I didn't have a sense of humor, I would long ago have committed suicide."
—Mahatma Gandhi

"Through humor, you can soften some of the worst blows that life delivers. And once you find laughter, no matter how painful your situation might be, you can survive it."
—Bill Cosby

"Good humor is one of the preservatives of our peace and tranquility."
—Thomas Jefferson

"Humor is the instinct for taking pain playfully."
—Max Eastman

Movies I watch when I feel blue:

I find that when I'm really feeling down, turning to an old favorite brightens my mood. If you are "up to" senseless comedy, but don't know where to start, here are my personal favorites.

Dumb and Dumber
Young Frankenstein
White Chicks

The Best of___, Saturday Night Live (SNL)
Wedding Singer
Pee-Wee Herman's Big Adventure

Anything can be funny, anywhere, in any situation

You must wonder how humor can be found in something as terrifying as MS. Read the following quote and be reminded that *it's possible to laugh* in situations worse than your own.

"My guess is that even people at Auschwitz were telling jokes. It's human nature to find the light in darkness somehow."

—Jon Stewart, host of Comedy Central's *The Daily Show*

Did God have anything to do with your MS?

Early after my diagnosis, I was asked if I thought God deliberately caused my MS. My answer was that, if He did, He probably had a special purpose in mind, and it was my job to figure out what that purpose was.

Well-meaning friends and family members often say, "We pray for you." A friend of mine has a lovely aunt who is a Catholic nun and graciously placed my name on the church Mass dedication list for inclusion in weekly prayer. I'd be a damn fool to deny any potential power of prayer to improve my health circumstances, but I have personally *never* asked God to rid me of MS. If I do pray, it is to be given strength to endure the challenges I bear from this *godforsaken* disease.

Science and faith toggle for position on my philosophical compass. I believe that praying "to be healed" is an academic oxymoron, as serious Darwin followers must consider prayer a waste of time and energy that would be better directed toward discovering the "missing link." Yet, with so much that occurs without logic, there *must be* a reason beyond our simple comprehension of everything. I am neither a theologian nor on the saints-in-waiting list, but I truly believe that there is a master plan that is out of our reach.

If He (or She) is truly a loving God, there must be a justifiable intention for giving me this physical handicap. Perhaps I am to be a prophet of determination, perseverance, and tolerance or maybe a beacon of understanding and an inspiration to those living in despair.

Whatever my role, I hope that I am able to perform even a small part with integrity. I have used any opportunity to teach others about MS—especially children, as they tend to be compassionate and most eager to learn. I may never know for certain if I have been successful, but I continue to reach out to people with a modest amount of encouragement by sharing the message, "Yes, you can do it."

Superman doesn't have superpowers anymore?

Christopher Reeve's entire life changed in a matter of seconds as he was competing in a horse-jumping tournament. Although Reeve is best remembered for playing Superman in the 1980s movie by the same name, he *was* Superman incarnate to many people around the world. All were saddened by his tragic accident and struggled to adjust to news of our hero's physical losses.

Christopher Reeve was completely paralyzed from head to toe; nonetheless, he always revealed a strong, healthy attitude. But what do you think made him such a seemingly content, pleasant, and positive man? Was it the scores of adoring fans across the globe who expressed their admiration and support? Was his contentment based on the love and support of his wife and son? The satisfaction and success he had accumulated during his professional years as an actor?

Probably, all of these elements influenced Reeve's attitude, but I contend the inner strength he gained was from giving hope to the hopeless—to those paralyzed with spinal-cord injuries. Christopher Reeve became a hero for all paraplegic and quadriplegic disabled persons by putting his celebrity power to productive and compassionate use. He dedicated his time, energy, and name to garner unprecedented interest in spinal-cord research around the world.

I can appreciate this, as I have personally experienced a sense of satisfaction from being able to share what I have learned about the physical, emotional, and social challenges I have faced with progressive MS.

How bad is bad? The young man with amputated legs

Blake Haxtun is a handsome, bright, former athletic high school crewmember. He was a senior from Upper Arlington High School when both of his legs were removed above the knee because of a runaway infection of necrotizing fasciitis. My son, who was supposed to graduate with Blake in June 2009, asked me whose disability I thought was worse—Blake's or mine.

Let's see: Blake's upper body and corporeal muscle were unaffected, but his disability caused a shocking, unexpected disruption to his relatively young life. My disability from MS had been slowly progressing for more than a decade. After some thought, I responded that I felt Blake had the "worse disability."

This tragic event happened to Blake when he was a mere eighteen-year-old *young* kid, while I was approaching fifty and had spent the majority of my adult years exploring different life experiences. Most important, I felt Blake's circumstance was sudden and alarming, whereas mine was gradual and expected. I could anticipate and prepare myself for forecasted changes.

There really is no easy way to answer this question, but perhaps the person who is "better off" is the one who has found a sense of peace, comfort, and strength to use his or her disabilities for a greater good.

"I shouldn't complain about my problems while you have MS!"

Some people stop dead in their tracks when they catch themselves complaining about a petty health ailment, compared to my physical dysfunctions from MS. I assure them that I do not find their complaint disrespectful and try to extinguish their embarrassment. I aim to convince them that even one simple, seemingly insignificant problem can become magnified into the central focus of one's life.

Mind over matter

Some annoyances in life can be hard to ignore and will test your resilience. If I need to scratch an itch or brush away an annoying bug, for example, and no one is around to help, I must force my mind to pay no attention. If I am in need of assistance, I often can't (and don't) ask for everything at one time as it is more efficient to "pick my battles," prioritize my complaints, and only ask for assistance to help with my greatest needs.

I remind myself that limitations because of my confined circumstances pale in comparison to others who have endured years of (possibly endless) captivity. Nelson Mandela spent twenty-seven years locked in a South African jail, and Sen. John McCain of Arizona, who was captured by the North Vietnamese in the Vietnam War, was a prisoner for five and a half years. With great concentration, I can apply the power of my mind to tolerate prolonged loneliness. I isolate my mind as the only "muscle" in my body and *convince* myself that my predicament has been solved. When I succeed, it is quite an accomplishment.

My resolve and patience should be credited to my Catholic upbringing. As a young student at a traditional Roman Catholic school, I was required to attend Mass every morning for an hour *before* classes began at 8 a.m. As a kid, sitting motionless in a pew for a boring sixty-minute Catholic Mass is torturous and requires you to occupy your mind to survive repeated text in the early morning, day after day. If those times didn't teach me the art of fortitude, nothing would.

Staying involved

In honor of the marriage of Prince William of Wales to Catherine Middleton, a group of girlfriends and I met for breakfast at a teahouse restaurant located in an old, wealthy neighborhood in Columbus. The interior of the venue lent an old English ambience, and the pristine menu included items such as white chocolate lavender scones and Swiss cheese quiche.

Another group of women who were also celebrating the "big wedding" sat down at the next table. All of us were wearing fashionable hats for the occasion. We gabbed about the order of marriages in the Royal Family and the proper definitions of low, afternoon, and high tea.

I didn't need to act like a member of British society to enjoy myself that day. Merely having this social opportunity allowed me to harness positive energy and combat the destruction caused by this ferocious disease. There are an infinite number of things to enjoy in life, and MS doesn't stop me from engaging in them.

Maintain exposure to a fun and exciting world around you, and don't let the MS devil win and take it all away.

He taketh away, but He giveth in return

Early on, I mourned the passing of what I had and what I did with it when I had it. But amazingly, my cognitive function was enhanced, which made my muscle failure a bit more tolerable and improved my acceptance of MS.

My sensory perception also became keener as my muscles failed me; so did my ability to identify sounds, tastes, thoughts, and emotions more vividly. I became more proficient at crafting my words and a better communicator with my facial expressions. Since I couldn't document and write information on paper, I coaxed myself to store more audio and video data in my memory.

At this point, I figure I'll take what I can get.

A little morale boosting goes a long way

I imagine each of us has experienced an instance where one person made a comment that changed our lives forever.

A delightful, vivacious neighbor and mother of eleven children gave me a much-needed morale boost during an impromptu conversation at our children's middle school. I have always held her in high esteem because she volunteers much of her time and energy to the church and to her children's schools in addition to raising a large family.

I was tickled and honored to be applauded by her for my tenacious spirit despite being a single mother with MS. Her compliments were heartfelt and intensely emotional, as she talked about her familiarity with the struggles of disability when she nurtured a daughter with cerebral palsy. Her words stifled my breathing. She is unaware that I credit her greatly for giving me the power to fight the fight, but she did just that.

A word from the late, great Mr. Rogers

I gained an insightful perspective on disability from the book *The World According to Mr. Rogers*, written by the beloved Fred Rogers from *Mister Rogers' Neighborhood*. This passage is from the chapter "The Courage to Be Yourself":

"Part of the problem with the word *disabilities* is that it immediately suggests an inability to see or hear or walk or do other things that many of us take for granted. But what of people who can't feel? Or talk about their feelings? Or manage their feelings in constructive ways? What of people who aren't able to form close and strong relationships? And people who cannot find fulfillment in their lives, or those who have lost hope, who lived in disappointment and bitterness and find in this life no joy, no love? These, it seems to me, are the real disabilities."

Wow. He may have hit the nail on the head.

Index